UNFORGETTABLE

UNFORGETTABLE

TRIBUTE TO OUR HEROES AND VICTIMS OF 9/11

SIMEON W. JOHNSON

ISBN: 979-8-3492-5951-7 (Paperback)
ISBN: 979-8-3492-5952-4 (eBook)

Printed in the United States of America

CONTENTS

EXCERPT

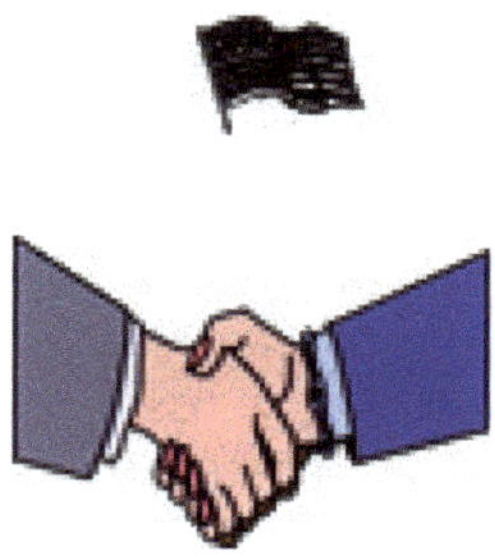

Unforgettable Tribute to our Nation's Finest and Bravest, and the Victims of 9/11

- In honor of our nation's finest bravest, and the victims of 9/11. The redoubtable firefighters and police officers who gave their lives to save others¾in light of the hideous assaults perpetrated on innocent individuals who lost their lives at the World Trade Center — now known as ground zero, on Tuesday, September 11, 2001.
- The etymology of the word "redoubtable" is defined by many noble words.

Redoubtable:

Widely known and honored for achievement, famous, celebrated, eminent, famed, great, notable, prominent, renowned, etc.

- As the eyes of the world saw your bravery and heroism as you gallantly gave your lives for others. In my opinion, it is a minor variance of word definition to lionize and honor you with the meritorious description of the above. Your stalwart demonstration of courage has placed you in the ranks of the redoubtable in light of your gallant act of altruism and heroic service to your fellowmen.
- Allow me to intersperse this illustrative anecdote: Julius Caesar's three-word pronouncement, Veni, Vidi, Vici ("I came, I saw, I conquered") is one of the most famous laconic statements of all time…

- With all due respect, however, the command given to Moses, to return to Egypt with the proclamation "I AM THAT I AM have sent you," supersedes the above statement.
- You were not able to say as Julius Caesar has said, "I came, I saw, I conquered", however, you came and saw the horrific scene... and heard the cacophony of sound emanating from those towering infernos of the World Trade Center... You conquered the fear of danger with alacrity, without fear of loosing your own lives in order to save others! You came, you saw, you conquered the fear of death, by saving many others! Your unselfish meritorious act of bravery has enriched us all.
- UNFORGETTABLE TRIBUTE TO OUR HEROES ***AND THE VICTIMS OF 9/11*** is a book essential for the events of the day, available through the Internet @ www.barnes&noble.com, www.buybooksontheweb.com,www.amazon.com, www.swjenterprise.com, or call Toll-Free (877) BUY BOOK.

- No. Of Pages: Approx. 130 Paperback ©

  US$ 10.95

  ISBN 0-7414-1013-3

  Publication Year, (2002)

  SIMEON W. JOHNSON

  From his book titled

  Unforgettable Tribute To Our Heroes and the Victims of 9/11

P.S. The following is a thank you note from former President Bill Clinton!

Thank you so much for your kind gift. I appreciate your thoughtfulness and generosity. You have my best wishes.

Bill Clinton

IN THIS BOOK, YOU'LL DISCOVER...

- The impact on our children after the events of September 11, ...
- **Abraham Lincoln,** twelve major failures before he was elected President of the United States at age 52
- **Ludwig van Beethoven,** triumph over his hearing loss and went on to...
- **Elizabeth Murray,** a teenager who went from living on the streets in New York City, to...
- **John Milton,** was blind at the age of 44, Sixteen years later he wrote...
- **Chester Carison,** in the 1940s, 20 corporations rejected his idea. His tiny company was bought and became Xerox Corporation.
- **Wilma Rudolph,** at the age of four, she contracted double pneumonia and scarlet fever, leaving her left leg paralyzed. Was told she would never walk again. She went on to win...
- **Clint Eastwood,** in 1959, Universal Pictures executive told him...
- **Lucille Ball,** in 1927, the head instructor of John Murray told her...
- **Elvis Presley** was told...
- **Albert Einstein** did not start speaking until he was...
- **Burt Reynolds,** in 1959, he was told...
- **General Douglass Macarthur,** he was denied...
- **Thomas Edison,** when he attended school, his teacher told him he was...
- **Arnold Schwarznegger** was told...
- **Colonel Sanders** was rejected 1,009 times before...
- **Beatrice Wood (artist),** experienced numerous failures, poverty and bad marriages before her success as...**...** Plus much, much more...

About the Author

Simeon W. Johnson is the author of ***Unforgettable Tribute To our Heroes and the Victims of 9/11 …*** His other books include ***Romw vs. Ramb, and A Myopic Life Resonated.*** Mr. Johnson has completed a Master's course in Radio TV Electronics. He earned his FCC General Radio Telephone First Class license with Radar endorsement. He currently lives and works in New York City and has appeared on numerous local and national radio shows.

Dedication

In honor of my Grandson Brian, and Granddaughter Amira
Welcome to life! Your birth has brought a
Plethora of refulgent happiness to your Grandma and me …
Like rising stars, I hope you will shine bright…
For yourselves and your parents! Most of all…
For the one in whose hands your future lies!

Love,
Grandma and Grandpa
Simeon and Dorothy Johnson

Simeon W. Johnson

Presents

Unforgettable Tribute to our Heroes and Victims of 9/11

RELIEF vs. STRESS

What This Book Will Do for You

It will reduce the stress level of every day chores, especially after the aftermath of September 11th. It is true however, the invention of modern conveniences has improved the lives of many: On the other hand, it has greatly increased the anxiety and stress levels of others in many ways.

The good news is, in this book you will discover a plethora of hopeful optimism, and a precipitous decrease in posttraumatic stress disorder.

United we stand against the access of evil…

"Words are the tools of thoughts by which men gather their thoughts and communicates with each other!" Therefore, it is within the context of this truism I chose to express my thoughts and reflections in the wake of September 11th, and the events of the day!

CHAPTER 1

UNFORGETTABLE TRIBUTE TO OUR HEROES AND VICTIMS OF 9/11

The unforgettable Tribute to our Heroes; and Victims of 9/11, clearly demonstrated [Alacrity vs. Celerity], which is the duty of every firefighter and law enforcement officer to answer the call of duty with alacrity, and eschew the lure of evil with celerity!

There are numerous examples throughout the annals of history that demonstrate this truism. Case in point: Here is a paragon example of Joseph's courageous act in the saga of his experience in Egypt as Potiphar's wife tempted him salaciously.

He eschewed precipitously, the lure of that effervescent temptation that startled him.

On that day in infamy when the most catastrophic act of terrorism took place in the history of the United States of America, hijackers took over a number of airplanes and, in a hideous act of suicide, they blew up the World Trade Center, located in New York City, taking the lives of thousands of innocent men, women, and children with them, and almost succeeded in blowing up our nation's Capital the seat of power of this great nation ... (Three thousand were lost in the WTC)

Nowhere has it been more demonstrable than in recent events in New York City and in our nation's Capital.

The firefighters answered the call of duty by rushing to the call of a fire alarm to save lives and property… the crime fighters race to the scene of a crime with fearless celerity as the drama unfolds.

With that said, however, in reality, "that is easier said than done" A police officer may rush to the scene of a crime, such as a hostage-taken situation, only to find him-or herself engaged in negotiations with the hostage taker. In this scenario, it requires a sagacious methodical plan of action, not a cursory reaction.

This is a fair assumption, that every able-bodied human being at some point in their lives had similar experiences, where the foregoing scenario has been played out in one way or the other.

This may be the case in our own family, as with sibling revelry… among adults. Brother against brother; sister against sister, children against parents, husband against wives… neighbor against neighbor, etc. With every contentious situation however, there can be a peaceful resolution to that crisis.

Human beings by nature have this God given ability to rationalize and settle their differences without reacting to impetuous negative impulse.

Realistically speaking, however, there are some calls to duty which may not be so inviting to our response, which we may find abhorrent to our conscience; such as premeditated murder; the act of capital punishment, etc.

There are many other characteristics of human traits, which we have the ability to rationalize before reacting to negative impetuous impulses.

Let us think of the many times in our lives that we acted on negative impulses instead of a methodical response.

Unlike the firefighter answering the call of duty with eagerness and cheerfulness to action… The crime fighter responding to the scene of a crime with celerity…

We walk across the street out of the way of speeding traffic with celerity. We answer the telephone of an anticipated call with eagerness or promptness; depending on the circumstances… It may be a favorable or unfavorable expectation: Nevertheless, we answer the call with [celerity], not knowing what to expect.

Case in point: Every spouse at one time or the other, whether at work or your places of leisure, have had a message of sorts, either from home, the hospital, the school principal, or school nurse, conveying a message vis-à-vis, good or bad. In this situation, you answer the call with swiftness of action or motion. In other situations, the call may be from a police officer telling you that your loved one is in jail due to a minor or major infraction of the law. This time you answer the call with celerity and apprehension! Not with cheerful readiness, eagerness, or promptness in action or movement as the firefighters duty to answer every alarm with alacrity!

The infamous events on September 11, 2001, in New York City and in Washington DC, at the Pentagon, where hundreds of deaths and injuries occurred by those hideous suicide bombers — is a vivid reminder of man's inhumanity to man; yet on the other side of man… there is an inborn desire to help our fellowman when the need arises. As demonstrated by those brave firefighters, police officers, and those Good Samaritans, who answered the call of duty with alacrity and, in addition, eschewed danger with celerity — underscores the true meaning of the words.

Personal Experience

Allow me to share this story . . . from my personal experience as a child: As a young child. I fell from a pimento tree and landed supine on my back! My neighbor, from a considerable distance away, heard the loud sound as I fell and lay prostrate.

My call for help went unanswered. Unfortunately, there were no EMS personnel to rush me to the hospital! The availability of

EMS service in a rustic community was not a viable convenient for a bucolic way of life! Something the urbane city dwellers take for granted.

Pimento, for example, is an expensive natural resource commonly grown in some areas of Jamaica, and when we were kids, we relied on the pimento harvest for spending money for the holiday seasons…

I experienced a similar incident as a child! This time I fell from a plum tree on my back. This incident also got no response. As usual, there was no EMS personal to respond to my call with alacrity. Such is the way of a bucolic country life.

In addition to the previous statements . . . I will continue to elaborate on the subject of alacrity vs. celerity, and the difference in similarity between these two words in their respective situation…

I vividly remember an incident as a teenager when I was a spectator at an outdoor pond where the neighborhood boys usually had unsupervised recreational swimming!

I was there as a spectator, not knowing how to swim, watching the boys as they enjoyed their swim! One of the boys jokingly came after me to throw me in the water . . . As the saying goes! "Boys will be boys."

He reached out to grab and pull me in the water! I sensed danger, and ran with celerity away from that imminent danger. Unlike [alacrity] cheerful readiness, eagerness, and promptness in action! This was obviously an imminent danger to eschew at all costs.

Even though I had a machete in my hand at the time of that incident... if I had not escaped, in retrospect, I probably would have committed an egregious offence in defense of my own protection. I ran with celerity for my life.

The Saga Continued

As I continue the saga of my youthful episode, at this time, there was another incident where my friends and I were in a large swimming pool of a very opulent camp near-by.

While I was standing in the water, not being able to swim, as I have stated before, one of my neighborhood friends recklessly dove over my head, and knocked my head down under the water where I almost drowned, after I swallowed much water.

As I regained consciousness with my machete in my hand… I ran with [celerity]: swiftness of action, and a thirst for revenge! I ran after my friend to execute vengeance on him.

That was a call to action with deadly force, unlike the firefighter's call to duty with promptness of action to save others!

Similar to the above incidents, a neighborhood bully provoked me to anger, but with quick mordent wit, and a clever twist of thought, I picked up a stone nearby, and threw it at him, hitting him in the ribs.

He curled up in pain from the blow he sustained! As I stood a safe distance away from him, commiserating with remorse over my action, wanting to have a [rapprochement], a peaceful reconciliation with him! I also made an earnest attempt to assuage the pain I inflicted on him, to no avail. As he regained strength, he came at me viciously. I ran with celerity from the imminent danger that ensued.

As I ran and sought refuge on the porch of the neighborhood preacher, he came out to investigate the commotion. Instead of praying for my deliverance from the truculent rage of my attacker, he was very phlegmatic about the whole incident; and escorted us off his porch into the street where we belonged!

While we were out on the street facing a difficult situation, instinctively, with mordant wit and clever twist of thought, I said to the person, "Would you pick up a stone and describe what happened?" Surprisingly, he did!

As he stooped down to pick up a stone, I seized on that crucial moment and ran precipitously down the street, all the way home, from the onslaught of my attacker.

Again I was faced with a similar situation in my early teens, being assaulted by an older person who provoked me to anger in like manner! I seized on that moment when he was not aware of my tactical defense. With a large stick I had in my hand, I hit the person as hard I could, then took off and ran all the way home from imminent danger.

Recent Experience

Not too long ago I was crossing a busy intersection of the Bronx in New York. Suddenly a car careened around the corner while I was crossing. I tried to get out of the way of imminent danger as fast as I could; I slid and fell while doing so!

If I had not fallen in my haste to get out of the way of the speeding car, my legs could have been crushed or, worse, I could have been killed.

With that said, however, despite the jovial, witty, funny, ***bold*** act, to be eschewed and not repeated … One day on a Tuesday afternoon, I prayed for deliverance and was delivered from that hostility to a life of eternal security.

I responded with alacrity to the call of duty in the service of the Lord on that faithful Tuesday afternoon in the year 1964.

Further explanations are written in my books titled A Myopic Life Resonated, and the book titled: Romw vs. Ramb. Based on the saga of my life and the stolid opposition to my faith, I aver its authenticity with absolute certainty.

Such an ineffable act of redemption can't be compared with an incubus or mercurial description of the iconoclastic critics.

Great Man of History Who Burned the Midnight Oil

CHAPTER 2

The Redoubtable Albert Einstein's Acmatic Breakthrough, & How It Applies to Us Today...

Without question the redoubtable Albert Einstein's theory of relativity was an Acmatic breakthrough! Perhaps not too many people would argue with that profound statement: on the other hand, though, he may have reached the acme of his accomplishment. If he had not surrendered his will to the omniscient wisdom of the Creator who made it possible for him to acquire such plethoric knowledge. In the eyes of the omniscient Creator...

He has not fully achieved his creative potentials; despite his scientific legacy that has remarkably shaped western civilization through the quantum leap in the area of science and engineering, that brought us to the 21st Century cutting-edge technology, producing such engineering marvels that we are now witnessing in our time.

We need to be cognizant that these scientific breakthroughs and engineering marvels that inspire man to explore space beyond Earth's boundaries, attempting to colonize space by building the International Space Station, did not come about because of his creative intellectual genius but, from the intelligent Creator that made all things.

Scientists and engineers need to be cognizant of the fact that the knowledge they acquired enabling them to reach beyond the frontier of Earth, attempting to colonize space, did not come about by their creative intellect; but from the omniscient wisdom that is unmatched, unequal, unparallel, and unrivalled, the only one who knows the exact number of every grain of sand on the seashore! He knows the number of hairs on our heads.

There is nothing secret that he does not know! Despite the various languages known to the linguists, lexicographers and etymologists, there is not a single person who can simultaneously interpret all languages. Yet, the superior intelligence of the omniscient — masters them all.

Every whisper, every word, every thought, is known by the omniscient Creator of all things. For example, the physical media we rely on to communicate and transmit these languages originate from the source of unlimited wisdom, knowledge and understanding that is unmatched, unrivaled, unequal and cannot be depleted by usage, or with time.

In addition, man, for the most part, relies totally on physical media [radio waves] and satellites for his means of communication that is reliable only as long as the ionosphere is not disrupted by solar flare activities in the Earth's atmosphere.

All these byproducts of the redoubtable Albert Einstein Acmatic achievements are without question, a remarkable accomplishment... though finite in comparison to the infinite wisdom, knowledge, and understanding of the omniscient.

Omniscient Wisdom

Albert Einstein and all the renowned scientists, engineers, and mathematicians have not been able to scratch the surface of the depth of the wisdom and knowledge of the infinite wisdom of the omniscient.

Solomon, the wisest man who ever lived, was inspired to write of the omniscient in the following manner:

"He is wise and full of wisdom" Wisdom only He alone possessed, declared in this wise man. "The LORD possessed me in the beginning of his way, before his works of old."

I was set up from everlasting, from the beginning, or ever the earth was" (Proverbs 8:22,23). (KJV)

With all due respect to the omnifarious readers: You owe it to yourself to be pensive about your accomplishments, and realize that where ever there is force or energy used to do work! There must be a power source.

We have learned in basic science and electronics, that in order to generate electricity. We must have a continuous current flow from a source! The moment the connection of continuous current flow is broken, we no longer have power and remain in darkness until we mend the broken connection back to the source of power.

Therefore, how is it that finite mortals, think that they can break out of their creative chrysalis to achieve the recognition they think they deserve to be autonomous of the infinite source of power, to generate their own finite power?

There are those individuals who think that the redoubtable Albert Einstein and the elite group of esoteric scientists and engineers who have reached the acme of their achievements, and have broken out of their creative chrysalis in order to gain the recognition they think they deserve, by reaching for the stars.

They have reached the age of leaving planet earth to colonize space, by building an International Space Station to conduct scientific experiments conceivable, only to the esoteric minds.

As I have stated before! It is empirically important to be pensive about your action, and not forget the basic science and physics¾that taught us that in order to have an uninterrupted current flow! You must have an unbroken connection of continuous current flow from the source of power.

Let us be cognizant of the fact that the only source of uninterrupted power supplies ever existed; is the connection between man and the omnipotent power source! When that connection is broken, you remain in darkness and in a state of limbo.

How to Mend the Broken Connection

How to mend the broken connection from the source of power is for the most part, not esoteric. All you and I have to do is to have a permanent series connected circuit directly to the authentic source of power.

Not a parallel connection, I might add! However, a series connection, because, in a parallel connection, there are more than one connection to and from the source, and that is a no-no when dealing with the omnipotent power of God.

In a series connected circuit, however, there is only one continuous path to the source. If broken, you have no power. Therefore, in order for you to be in direct contact with the source, you need to mend the broken path by bridging the gap, in order to reestablish the unbroken link back to the source of power.

This, however, is the time to emphasize the relevancy of power in the diurnal of everyday life. Not even in the primitive and bucolic way of life, can anyone survive without some source of power. Whether it's a natural energy generated from the body or by artificial means, all sources of energy originate from the omnipotent and infinite source of power.

The heat generated by the penguins of the Antarctic during the inclement winter months, as they cuddle together, originates from the infinite source of power provided by the omnipotent provider and giver of life.

Man, for the most part, has flaunted his God-given ability to harness energy from various sources in order to keep our modern sophisticated way of life energized, and always on the cutting edge of high technology.

The parallel branch to and from the source from which man obtains his power — consists of many branches. However, this source from which man gets his power is the antithesis of what is required to harness his power from the ultimate powerhouse: The power of the most high.

Unlike the parallel path, however, which consist of many paths to the source of power. The unbroken path to the kingdom power is the only connection between man and the Creator of this infinite source of power.

Let us take, for example your Christmas decoration lights during the holiday seasons! If either one of those lights goes out, there are many other paths for current to flow from the source of power. The rest of the decorative lights remain active.

Likewise, the lights in your homes or apartments and places of business doesn't all go out at the same time, because they are parallel connected, having many paths to each fixtures! Unless of course there is a power surge that blew the main fuse or tripped the main circuit breaker.

This is not so, however, with a series circuit source! Whenever the only path to the circuit is broken, you will find yourself in the dark until the broken path is fixed.

This illustration intersperses my effort in focusing the refulgent beam of my candlelight on the path to the kingdom, so that others who stumble in darkness, seeking many paths, may focus on one path that lights the way to the powerhouse of infinite supply of power.

There are those who would argue that there are many ways to the Kingdom. In light of the foregoing examples however, all one has to do is to review the descriptive analyses of basic Science and Electricity, and decide for yourself whether the statement is true or not.

It is obvious that even a small peccadillo can interrupt the flow of a series connection with the source of infinite power. A classic example are our first parents, who broke the original series connection to the infinite Power

Supply to their Creator. Henceforth, the potential for power outage has plagued the human race ever since.

The unbroken connections between man and his Creator was broken because of disobedience, and because of that broken connection! The ubiquitous presence of sin pervades the hearts of men and women everywhere.

The good news is, however, "Where sin abounded, grace did much more abound:" (Romans 5:20) (KJV)

Allow me to interject this tangential discussion, though not exactly related to the subject matter. Nevertheless:

During the events of September 11, at the World Trade Center in New York City, in the state of Pennsylvania, and in Washington, at the Pentagon, there was a colloquial discussion on one of the major TV networks, the guests were asked of the survivability of the Theater District in New York City.

One of the guests responded by saying: " . . . Yes, the theater preceded religion as a necessity for mankind." My immediate reaction to the above quote inveigh this sharp retort in response!

In light of recent events, a person does not have to be of a religious persuasion to refute such a vain statement. The premise of the question makes the answer null and void. Allow me to illustrate the point. If the theater precedes religion as a necessity for humankind, why were churches filled to standing-room only after the September 11, attack?

Let us consider the question about the survivability of the vacant Theater District after the attack . . . Do you recall that, while the churches were filled to standing room only, we did not hear a national call for the theaters to open their doors for prayer and consolation.

Therefore, in response to the quote in question: “The theater preceded religion as a necessity for mankind.” The answer is: True religion will outlast the theater as a necessity for humankind, now and forever.

Allow me to interject the following epigraph from the redoubtable Albert Einstein.

“When the Special Theory of Relativity began to germinate in me, I was visited by all sorts of nervous conflicts… I used to go away for weeks in a state of confusion.”

Einstein reported a remarkable consequence of his special theory of relativity: “If a body emits a certain amount of energy, then the mass of that body must decrease by a proportionate amount.’ Meanwhile he wrote a friend, “The relativity principle in connection with the Maxwell equations demands the mass is a direct measure for the energy contained in bodies; light transfers mass… This thought is amusing and infectious, but I cannot possibly know whether the good Lord does not laugh at it and has led me up the garden path.” ‘Einstein and many others were soon convinced of its truth.’ The relationship is expressed as an equation: $E=mc^2$.

With all due respect to the redoubtable Albert Einstein and associates, your esoteric theory and formula of relativity may be right in the realm of Science and Physics, but not so with the infinite source of power emanating from the Omnipotent, which is inexhaustible, unparallel, unrivaled and unequal, and cannot be depleted with time or usage.

Albert Einstein was blessed with the gift of an esoteric, erudite mind, but was not known to speak with a terse mordant wit and trenchant retort!

CHAPTER 3

How to Deal with Transient Failures

How to deal with transient failures is a common concern among human beings. One of the first rules however, is to act as if it was impossible to fail, and you will always succeed!

The events on September 11, are a classic example of the inborn desire mankind has to succeed in spite of the overwhelming odds we face in the vicissitudes of daily life.

Never before in our time have we seen such resilience in the willingness of the people of this great country to rally around a cause to form a common bond in helping one another, and a desire to seek the help of a higher Power than ourselves...

We witnessed the hideous assault perpetrated on the people in the World Trade Center and our nation as a whole, and the reckless disregard for human life by the hateful and detestable act of those terrorists.

Though it might appear otherwise our City's finest and bravest have failed in their efforts to save everyone. Their heroic effort has left us a rich legacy of true altruism.

This is an important lesson you have taught us: that giving of oneself in order to save others can serve as a paragon example to follow!

Notice that, out of the dark ruins of ashes and debris of this disaster, resulted a resonance of spiritual awakening the likes of which this nation has never seen in recent memory.

Never in the history of this nation, have we seen such a venerable display of patriotism and spiritual awaking, where humankind sought the help of a higher power through the medium of prayer.

We have demonstrated that we are a nation whose motto is, "In God we trust" though we have strayed from the old path. For the most part, we still believe "prayer changes things," especially in times of crisis. Therefore, failure is not an option we have chosen in our effort to rebuild after September 11, 2001.

To all those who have contributed to the noble cause of helping others, especially for such a worthy cause in this time of tremendous loss and hurt, your works and labor of love will make a difference to those whose lives you have touched.

Your philanthropic outpouring of love and compassion for your fellowmen demonstrates Alacrity. Cheerfulness of action to help: vs. Celerity. Swiftness of action to tear down, kill and destroy!

Rising to the occasion

With God's help, America will rise again to continue its task to defend its sovereignty and maintain its role as a leader of the free world.

History has taught us that out of evil or natural disaster good things can happen. The most recent proof of this profound statement is the September 11, World Trade Center disaster, and the aftermath of a spiritual resonance that America has not seen in recent memory.

In Biblical times, the Prophet Nehemiah heard of the destruction of the wall of the City of Jerusalem... He did not accede! Instead, with God's help; he rebuilt the wall of the City— demonstrating vigilance as he rebuilt... with a sword in one hand, and the tool of his craft in the other hand, while others served as watchmen... all served in unison in their own capacity (Nehemiah 4: 17).

We can learn from this event in history as America begins its rebuilding process, with God's help, of course, while at the same time be on its guard against the enemy of a free and open society, not letting down its guard, yet being prepared to protect its interest both at home and around the world.

Turning Failure into Triumph

Turning failure into triumph can be an arduous task to accomplish, in light of what our nation and the world has come to realize since the incidents of September 11, 2001.

In the eyes of the critics, some would see this as failure to follow up on leads that could have averted this disaster. America did not capitulate nor accede to the terrorist demands. We learned from our failures, and are taking measures to prevent similar incidents from happening again.

That our nation is fighting the enemy to put an end to this terrorism madness, at the same time beefing up national and local security, shows that we have learned from our failures, and the results are unprecedented steps taken to prevent this type of disaster from recurring.

After eyewitness accounts of the horrific disaster on September 11, at New York City's World Trade Center; Washington, D.C. at the Pentagon, and Pennsylvania, we have taken extraordinary steps to insure public safety and restore confidence in the minds of the people everywhere; we are more vigilant than we were before.

All these measures are a direct result of turning failures into triumph! Surveys show that on the Sunday following the horrific disaster, over ninety Percent of church attendance was standing room only.

This brings to memory, the words of the Prophet Ezekiel, which reads:

"But if the watchman sees the sword come, and blow not the trumpet, and the people be not warned; if the sword come, and take any person from among them, he is taken away in his iniquity; but his blood will I require at the watchman's hand" (Ezekiel 33:6).

Brief description prior to the events of September 11, are explained in Chapter 9 of my book titled A Myopic Life Resonated, Published July 1998. Re-published June 2001.

With that said allow me to change the venue of the subject matter without being tangential— to the vicissitude of everyday life that touch us individually.

Behind Every Successful Story

Permit me to coin this truism, that behind every successful story, there are a myriad of failures. The events of September 11 give us a panoramic view of what life in America is like… It shows that in a moment's time, a life can be changed from one stage to the next… for better or for worse.

For example, the successes and failures of great achievers that grace the covers of Fortune Five Hundred and Forbes Magazines, richest people in the world all had their failures prior to achieving their success with the exception of a few, of course.

By studying the history of the CEOs and owners of these fortune five hundred corporations: you will learn that these individuals did not start out rich and famous, with the exception of those individuals who inherited wealth.

Here are some sobering reminders of great men and women who have beaten the odds, have risen from humble beginnings, from rags to riches, and entered the ranks of the rich and famous.

- Two American Entrepreneurs: Madame C.J. Walker and , J.C. Penney overcame great odds and moved from ***rags*** to ***riches***
- "Madame C.J. Walker Building" and "J.C. Penney Historic District," Indianapolis (Indiana) site of Madame Walker's cosmetics business...
- The building is a four-story brick structure completed in 1927... Another building a thousand miles west of Indiana in Kemmerer, Wyoming, was the site of J.C. Penney's first department store; these two historic buildings provide insight into both characters of this country's most famous business people: Madame Walker and J.C. Penney overcame great odds, and both combined a desire to serve with great success...

Other stories of rags to riches are:

- Apple Computers
- Sears
- The Dow Jones Index and the Wall Street Journal
- Hershey's chocolate
- Kinney shoes
- Ebony magazine

These individual companies are just a few of many rags to riches stories we have known... They all burned the midnight oil, pursuing their dreams despite the vicissitude of everyday life trials and errors. Nevertheless, they overcame the odds... We owe it to ourselves to gain from the successes of these stories.

Now that we have covered a few of many rags to riches stories of the common people, allow me to turn your attention to individuals like the redoubtable Albert Einstein: Despite his erudite intellect, we know, according to family legend, that he was a slow talker at first, pausing to consider what he would say.

Although he got generally good grades (and was outstanding in mathematics), Einstein hated the academic high school he attended in Munich, where success depended on memorizing and obedience to authority. His real studies were at home with books on mathematics, physics, and philosophy. A teacher suggested Einstein leave school, since his very presence destroyed the other students respect for the teacher. At the age of fifteen, he quit school in mid-term to join his parents, who had moved to Italy.

In 1895, Einstein failed an examination that, after a number of false starts, confirmed his predictions.

Einstein failed an entrance exam to secondary school! Original from, Einstein's general relativity, verified numerous times in the overview of his life, from childhood through the final decades of his life.

How Einstein Overcame Failures

Albert Einstein did not start speaking until he was four. He … failed the entrance exam to a university a number of times — and made his great discoveries after many failures.

Following are quotes from the erudite intellect of the redoubtable Albert Einstein

"If something great failed you, does it follow… be realized an infinite number of times. And since between… Law and order" —Albert Einstein, letter to Max…

"There was this huge world out there, independent of us human beings and standing before us like a great, eternal, at least partly accessible to our inspection and thought. The contemplation of that world beckoned like a liberation."

Formative Years

"It is almost a miracle that modern teaching methods have not yet entirely strangled the holy curiosity of inquiry; for what this delicate little plant needs more than anything, besides stimulation, is freedom."

Einstein's family had moved to Italy to try to establish a business, and he joined them for a glorious half year of freedom from work and anxiety. In 1895, he took the entrance examination for the Swiss Federal Institute of Technology — he failed. He studied at Swiss School in Arau; here his teachers were humane and his ideas were set free. His thoughts turned to the theory of electromagnetism formulated by James Clark Maxwell, seldom taught even in universities at the turn of the century.

Meeting the Challenges

Now that we've learned of failures and successes of the rich and famous… Allow me to address the many failures and successes in our own lives. How often you and I as individuals encounter some of lives daunting problems?

The vicissitudes of daily life is one continuous challenge after the other! As soon as one problem is passed and those cherished moments of short-lived victory begin to materialize, we have a tendency to let down our guard…

Suddenly we are hit with another situation that robes us of that short-lived victory.

The question now is: How do we face these new challenges head on without resorting to negative feelings of bitterness and resentment?

We need to stay focused by saying to ourselves: This too will pass! Yesterday's problem is history [transient]. "Yesterday's passed, and tomorrow may never be mine!" I will deal with each issue one at a time.

Remember that situation in your life, which you thought was the straw that breaks the camel's back. Did it really? After all, you are still here to talk about it, are you not? With the same help of providence, you have solved your previous problems. With similar help, you will be able to solve many of life's problems.

That is easer said than done, you may be saying in your mind: How about those people who are suffering all the time? The young, the old and the infirm... Without question, that may be so.

What would you rather do? Contend with the hands of providence or be thankful and courageous in every adverse situation, whether trivial or life threatening? After all, your arm is too short to box with God.

It is better to have a rapprochement with the giver of life, than to be contentious... Contention leads to resentments and bitterness, and that does not play well with the one who holds your life and future in his hands.

The previous examples of the rise of ordinary, everyday people to world-renowned men and women of Acmatic achievers, who have worked tirelessly in their pursuit of fame and fortune to reach success in life, were not quitters but winners!

It is not easy to be optimistic all the time, especially when you know the situation of life is one continuous challenge after the other, from within as well as from without.

The challenges from within can be one's own negative fear of failure, such as what if I try at something and fail? What would people think of me, you might ask in reply to your question. You may think no good of yourself. The answer should be: "Greater is the power in me to succeed than the fear of those who have nothing to fear but phobophobia: fear itself.

The life story of great men and women who have succeeded in life is an open book of many failures through trials and errors they have experienced. Nevertheless, that did not thwart their God-given ability to be resilient, with fortitude and determination to succeed... Now, I will end this chapter with some sobering thought.

HOPEFUL OPTIMISM

The most successful failures... People who were told they would never succeed!

This page is a dedication to those faced with great obstacles in the vicissitudes of daily life! Remember the words of the Author of perfection..."Perfect love casts out all fear" ... Also, remember, the old saying. " The only thing we have to fear is fear itself"

Abraham Lincoln

- He entered the Black Hawk War as a captain. By the end of the war, he had been demoted to the ranks of private.
- Failed in business at age 21
- Defeated in a legislative race at age 22
- Failed again in business at age 24
- Overcame the death of his sweetheart at age 26
- Had a nervous breakdown at age 27
- Lost a congressional race at age 34
- Lost a congressional race at age 36

- Lost a senatorial race at age 45
- Failed in an effort to become vice-president at age 47
- Lost a senatorial race at age 49
- Was elected President of the United States at age 52

Ludwig van Beethoven

- By age 46 was completely deaf after progressive hearing loss. Nevertheless, he wrote his greatest music including five symphonies, during his later years.

Billy Joel

- His high school diploma was denied due to excessive absenteeism, ran away from home, and was arrested on alleged burglary… The charges were dropped, but a terrifying night in jail did little to build a happy outlook on life…
- He attempted suicide by drinking furniture polish.
- When that didn't solve the problem, he committed himself to the mental ward at Meadowbrook Hospital for three weeks observation and quickly discovered that he was quite sane.

  The hospital visit strengthened his resolve to make it in rock and roll: He had many more failures until he finally succeeded.

Elizabeth Murray

- A teenager who went from living on the streets in New York City to Harvard University — and is said to have worked for the New York Times…

Buddy Holly

- In 1956, Paul Cohen fired him from the Decca Recording Co. and called Holly "the biggest no-talent I ever worked with."

John Milton

- Was blind at the age of 44. Sixteen years later, he wrote Paradise Lost

Chester Carison

- In the 1940s, 20 corporations rejected his idea.

  After seven long years of rejections, a tiny company called the Haloid Company purchased the rights to his electrostatic paper-copying process: Haloid became Xerox Corporation

Wilma Rudolph

- At the age of four, she contracted double pneumonia and scarlet fever, leaving her left leg paralyzed. Her mother was told she would never walk again. She removed her metal brace by age nine and by age 13 she had developed a rhythmic walk: at the same time she decided to become a runner: She entered every race and came in last. Every- one told her to quit, but she kept on running until one day she actually won a race. From then on, she won every race. In addition, she went on to win three Olympic gold medals.

Clint Eastwood

- In 1959, an Universal Pictures executive told him that he had a chip on his tooth and his Adam's apple sticks out too far. In addition, he talked too slowly.

Lucille Ball

- In 1927, the head instructor of John Murray Anderson Drama School told her, "Try any other profession. Any other."

Elvis Presley

- Was told "You aren't goin' nowhere … son. You ought to go back to driving a truck."

Burt Reynolds

- In 1959 was told by a Universal Pictures executive that he had no talent.

Albert Einstein

- Did not start speaking until he was four years old: There was even some concern on the part of his parents when he was a young child that he might be somewhat backward! During his school years, he showed no special aptitude. In addition, because of his dislike of rigid methods of school officials cited him as being disruptive.

  He failed the entrance exam to a university a number of times and made his great discoveries while working by day in a low-level clerical job, … many today say that he was dyslexic.

General Douglas Macarthur

- He was turned down admission to West Point two times. He was finally accepted on his third attempt.

Thomas Edison

- When he first attended school his teachers complained he was "too slow" and hard to handle. He tried over 2,000 experiments before he got the light bulb to work.

Arnold Schwarznegger

- Was told if he wanted to succeed as an actor he better learn to speak without an accent and change his name.

Woody Allen

- Failed Motion Picture Production and English at New York University.

Colonel Sanders

- Was rejected 1,009 times before someone would back his business. He started Kentucky Fried Chicken.

Jim Carrey

- When he was teenager, he and his family were janitors at Titan Wheels and they lived in a tent on their aunt's lawn.
- **Comedy Club:** He bombed big time. Two years later Jim returned to Yuk Yuk and was great.

Al Pacino

- Got rejected for the part of Michael in "The
- Godfather" a number of times before he won the role…

Beatrice Wood (artist)

- She experienced numerous failures, poverty and bad marriages before her success as an artist later in life¾she is the inspiration for Katherine in the novel "Jules et Jim" and for the older Rose in the film "Titanic" (details are outlined in her autobiography "I Shock Myself").

With that said, however, and the plethora of information provided those who tirelessly burn the midnight oil through laborious effort, enabling them to break out of their creative chrysalis to achieve their purpose in life.

Unfortunately for many… that purpose may be transient, unlike that of the patriarch Abraham, who sought a dwelling place "whose builder and maker is everlasting."

We owe it to ourselves to embrace hopeful optimism with Alacrity! In addition, eschew the fear of failure with Celerity.

HOW TO DEAL WITH DEPRESSION
&
REJECTIONS

CHAPTER 4

How to Deal with Depression & Rejections

From a nonprofessional's point of view, one does not need a psychiatrist in order to deal with the daily nuances in life! If that weren't the case, everyone would have a psychiatrist. No one is immune from the vicissitudes of daily life.

Each individual situation is unique, requiring special attention in the need for professional care. With those exceptions, however, the rest of society needs a methodical approach in dealing with the inclement nuances of life.

There Are Many Kinds of Depression

Some depression is so banal in nature; it does not require the attention of a psychiatrist or professional counselor in order to deal with the situation. However, there are other kinds of depression that are more problematic to a degree — manic depression definitely has a deleterious effect on people's lives.

For example, the infamous events of September 11, at the World Trade Center, at the Pentagon and Pennsylvania, have created such a deleterious effect on the lives of so many people. The survivors who were at ground zero and the rest of civilize society, near and far, who were directly affected, may be experiencing a state of transient depression.

It has been reported that some victims of the hideous act perpetrated on America on September 11 are now suffering from recurring memories of those incredible events, including sleepless nights, anxiety and post traumatic stress syndrome.

Other visible signs of depression include sadness, feeling down in the dump, discouragement: the future looks hopeless!

Self-criticism and blaming yourself for everything ... Indecisiveness: having trouble making up your mind about things. Irritability and frustration, feeling resentful and angry most of the time…

Loss of motivation: feeling overwhelmed and having to push yourself hard to do things… your appetite may change, causing you to overeat… on the other hand, to not eat properly.

In light of recent events, you may be the guardian of your 15-year-old niece; she's a sophomore on the junior- varsity volleyball team. At the beginning of the season, she showed such adroit athletic ability that her coach considered moving her up the varsity team.

Recently, however, the coach has grown alarmed because her interest and enthusiasm for the sport has waned. She frequently misses practice and shows up late for games. The coach also notices she has lost some weight and is irritable. He asks if something is troubling her. She says yes. "I feel very lonely. My parents died on September 11, in one of the twin towers of the World Trade Center. They were always there for me whenever I had a problem."

In addition to the results of recent events, let us consider, for example, your-eight year-old nephew, who is always on the verge of tears, especially during the school day. Although he is normally a motivated student, his schoolwork is now suffering. Even at his young age, he understands the social stigma attached to boys who cry so he does his best to conceal his tears. His teacher notices him quietly crying one morning and asks what is wrong. " My parents have died and I'm very sad," he says.

Although these two young people are different genders and ages, both exhibit signs of depression. The popular belief that youths have jovial carefree childhood is not always the case.

Researchers indicate that, like adults, children experience depression in varying degrees. According to Dr. Michael Sorter, a psychiatrist at the Children's Hospital Medical Center in Cincinnati, Ohio, approximately five percent of adolescents experience depression. "We're talking about a large number of kids," he notes.

Much of this depression, unfortunately, is unrecognized and therefore untreated. Like depressed adults, however, children need loving support from others in order to overcome feelings of depression.

Cause and Effect of Depression

Other factors that can cause depression in a child or adults include:

- Moving to a new neighborhood
- Separation or divorce
- Remarriage and adjustment to a blended family
- Death of a family member, friend or even a pet
- Starting in a different school

Recognize the symptoms of depression: "Even the best parents can miss the signs of depression in children because they are distracted and preoccupied with their careers, marriages or daily parenting tasks. To avoid missing important clues, train yourself to recognize the following symptoms of depression listed by the National Institute of Mental Health (NIMH)."

- A persistent sad, empty or anxious mode
- Loss of interest or pleasure in ordinary activities
- Decreased energy or fatigue
- Sleep disturbance such as insomnia, early waking or oversleeping
- Difficulty concentrating or remembering
- Feeling of pessimism
- Chronic aches and pains that do not respond to treatment

Expert recommendation:

In his book, Stephen Merson, M.D., offers this advice; " Pretending there is not a problem is not an effective response, since the problem is likely to remain. Equally, it is important to avoid reacting in a negative fashion to a depressed individual.

"The first step must be to encourage the person to describe their situation. The most effective way of doing so is through patient and sympathetic listening that allows painful sentiments to be voiced. Make it clear that you are available and willing to help."

Encourage physical activity

Various studies demonstrate that regular exercise, produce above-normal levels of beta-endorphin, the body's natural hormone that increases pain tolerance and generally improves a person's mood. Enroll the child in team sports or at least suggest the child engage in some form of daily exercise, whether it is bicycling, jogging, swimming or walking. If the child is young, offer to join them in daily exercise routine.

In addition to the benefits of physical activity, the time together provides an excellent opportunity to discuss and explore feelings... [A personal note] Most paramount of all recommendations is the introduction to spiritual counseling.

Encourage friendship

Although depressed children often withdraw from family and friends, do whatever possible to encourage them to maintain contact with others… Friendships not only fill lonely hours but also prevent a depressed child from feeling completely alone and different. Friendship also generates healthy feelings of love and acceptance and offer crucial support to a person in emotional crisis.

People in emotional crisis

A recent study of 3,600 teens by the University of Minnesota Medical School revealed that young people seriously troubled by depression are much more likely to turn to their friends before they will talk to an adult. Of other teens involved in the study, more than a third felt depressed and 5.5 percent had attempted suicide in the past six months. Out of 54 possible coping-choices, talking with Mother was 31st, talking to Dad 48th and talking with a teacher, guidance counselor, clergy member or professional all tied for last place. The lesson learned from this study for caring adults: encourage a depressed child to spend time with their friends and suggest they invite companions to the house on weekends or after school.

Recommended ways of releasing feelings

New York psychiatrist Helen De Rosis advises young people to "Cry, pound pillows and complain to friends who can take it. This is a safe way to permit feelings of anger to surface. Anger is a very important part of depression and unless these angry feelings are released in some way, it is difficult to overcome depression."

Another effective way for young people to alleviate depression is by keeping a journal or diary in which feelings are noted. Write what you do and how you feel about all of this, Dr. De Rosis urges young people. "Ask yourself what impossible expectations you were trying to meet when you began to feel depressed. If an answer does not occur to you right away, do not worry. You may think of it a few days later."

Stimulate positive thinking

Youngsters with a tendency to become depressed think negatively, notes Douglass H. Powell, Ed. D., in his book. "They are obsessed about what's wrong with their lives, overestimate their flaws and underestimate their positive attributes, believe they can't do anything about them and think that everyone is as focused on their imperfection as they are." Dr. Powell advises caring adults to help youths identify the positives taking place in their lives on almost a daily basis, such as a good grade on a report card, a pleasant conversation with a friend, a compliment given by a teacher, the completion of a difficult task, etc.

Finally, parents should not compound youth depression by feeling guilty. Rather than blame yourself, praise yourself for recognizing it and for taking steps to correct your child's depression.

Victor M. Parachin is a National Funeral Directors

Association grief counselor and minister in Tulsa, OK.

Send comments and questions to vparachin@email.msn.com

Personal summation

The solution to the problem is not to let this brief period of depression consume you. In reality, do not deny your feelings of grief during this period of bereavement and reflection. If spiritual and professional help is not readily available to you while you are in a quandary, encourage yourself by saying: This too will pass. Be thankful for the opportunity of being alive.

Think of those who never made it out of those towering infernos alive, despite the magnanimous acts of altruism by New York's fire fighters, police officers and good samaritans who gave their lives to save others, answered the call of duty with Alacrity by cheerfully rushing into those burning buildings, not thinking of the danger they faced.

No one put a gun to their heads and forced them into those burning buildings. Each of those fire fighters, and police officers knew what they were getting into. They did not eschew danger with Celerity by running away from danger. On the other hand, they gave their lives with Alacrity, trying to save others. This is a classic example of true altruism.

With that said, the following statement illustrates the difference between finite love, and infinite love: "Greater love hath no man than this, that a man lay down his life for his friends" (John 15:13).

That is truly the ultimate love, unequal, unraveled, unmatched, a perfect example of true love that we should seek, as those heroic fire fighters and police officers demonstrated. When you and I experience periods of depression in our lives, let us consider the act of perfect love and not be defeated by periods of transient depression.

CHAPTER 5

DEALING WITH REJECTIONS

The preceding chapter deals with the cause and effect of depression. In this chapter, I will expatiate on the cause and effect of rejection!

The vicissitudes of daily life is one continuous challenge after another; therefore I will proceed with a subject that is tantamount to depression, the subject of rejections.

For example, if you fail an important subject, examination or test, that transient state of failure and rejection may cause you to sink to the nadir of your self- esteem, making you feel rejected and less important about yourself, thinking everyone is smarter than you are.

In such cases it does not require a psychiatrist to describe your feelings, which may be a normal reaction to the vicissitudes of life's daily challenges.

One way to deal with this reflective state of mind is not to ruminate over this transient setback in life, but rise to the occasion, regain your self-esteem by thinking of your recent triumphs. Encourage yourself, demonstrate a positive attitude, affirming that you are a worthwhile person, and it doesn't matter what people say or think of you.

When a negative feeling urges you to think of the failures in your life, do not dwell on this transient state of mind: Say to yourself. This too will pass… the next time I face this situation I will do better. If you choose the negative path, however, you will find yourself in a sullen state of mind, ruminating over the situation for a very long time.

Such a negative state will lead to depression of a deleterious nature.

There are many ways that a person can experience rejection. Case in point: Anyone who writes a book for the first time, knows what it feels like to be rejected by an agent or a publisher with the usual response, such as: Thank you for your interest in having us publish your book. However, it does not meet our requirements at this time.

Not only does this apply to a first-time writer, many seasoned writers can attest to similar rejections. Such cases do not always require the aid of a therapist.

Surveys show that, of the tens of thousands of books printed in the United States each year, only a small percentage gets published. Such statistics are very discouraging to an aspiring first-time writer; which is not a feeling of Alacrity to the one who experiences it¾yet life must go on.

Facing the Challenge

You can deal with the feeling of rejection and anxiety by turning a tragic situation into triumph; not letting rejection dictate your life. Say to yourself: I will not let an individual, negative opinion of me suppress my God-given potentials.

With the help of the "I AM THAT I AM" and with much fortitude and a considerable amount of mental gymnastics, I will break out of my creative chrysalis to achieve the recognition I deserve.

Many of history's best selling authors have had their first novel rejected many times by publishers before their work was finally accepted, and went on to become best sellers.

Rejections are not applicable only to aspiring authors, but to all human beings: therefore, you and I are not alone in these daily nuances of life.

When you believe your struggle is uniquely unfair, take comfort in knowing that the only perfect person who ever lived suffered the greatest rejection of all! Not because of any failures on his part — he was perfect in all his ways and the ways the Father. His rejection was by the myopic elite rulers of his day.

Most people have experienced rejections of one form or the other! Some rejections are very blatant while others are not. Nevertheless, all rejections, if not dealt with carefully can have a deleterious effect on your self-esteem.

Despite the excoriating hurt, most is not life threatening. Therefore, for those who have within their power to take control of the situation, let us move on without carrying the stigma of rejection on our shoulders for the rest of our lives.

Those brave and courageous civil rights leaders, who withstood the evil excoriation of discrimination and rejections, have brought inevitable change in this country and the world at large. Their peripatetic activism was not an act in futility but true altruism.

Rejection Is Experienced by All Races

Rejection is an indignity experienced by all, especially by the black minority! However, that is not a prerequisite that charts the course of our destiny. If that were the case, the black minority would be living in a state of onerous quandary about us.

If history has taught us anything, it has taught us that any-able bodied individual, if given an equal opportunity and a level playing field, can make a difference in this world!

Time and paper would not permit me to write of all the successful men, women, and all the minority communities and their contributions toward building a better society!

At this time however, I will attempt to expatiate on a few of the meritorious contributions of black America's contributions towards the building of this great nation, despite the insurmountable experiences of rejection.

The following epigraph is a testament of fact.

"Once let the black man get upon his person the brass letters, U.S., let him get an eagle on his button, and a musket on his shoulder and bullets in his pockets, and there is no power on earth which can deny that he has earned the right to citizenship in the United States."

Frederick Douglass

If all the black people in this country and the world at large — had acceded to the xenophobic rejections we have experienced throughout history had surrender their inalienable right? We would not have had the caliber of great pioneers, such as the Honorable Marcus Moriah Garvey, one of the greatest leaders of the African world, and the late Dr. Martin Luther King Jr., whose affinity for the oppressed of society, and many others who made such meritorious contributions for the cause of freedom and justice that enriched us all.

Those brave and courageous Civil Rights leaders, who withstood the evil excoriation of discrimination and rejections, have brought inevitable change in this country and the world at large. Their peripatetic activism was not an act in futility but true altruism.

History of African-Americans in the Civil War

The inspiring words spoken by Fredrick Douglass moved many African-Americans to enlist in the Union Army and fight for their freedom. After the Emancipation Proclamation in 1862, by President Abraham Lincoln, the Civil War became a war to save the union and to abolish slavery.

Approximately, 180,000 African-Americans comprising 163 units, served in the Union Army during the Civil War and many more African-Americans served in the Union Navy. Both free African-Americans and runaway slaves joined the fight.

On July 17, 1862, Congress passed two acts allowing the enlistment of African-Americans, but official enrollment occurred only after the September, 1862, issuance of the Emancipation Proclamation. In general, opposing soldiers and officers believed that black men lacked the courage to fight and fight well.

The Battle of New Market Heights, Virginia (Chaffin's Farm), became one of the most heroic engagements involving African-Americans. On September 29, 1864, the African-American division of the Eighteenth Corps, after being pinned down by confederate artillery fire for about 30 minutes, charged the earthworks and rushed up the slopes of the heights. During the hour-long engagement, the division suffered tremendous casualties. Sixteen African- Americans were awarded the Medal of Honor during the Civil War; fourteen received the honor because of their actions at New Market Heights.

Gallant meritorious act Tuskegee Airmen of World War II

In addition to the contributions of the black soldiers of the American Civil War era, during World War II: the Tuskegee Airmen made a major contribution. Where did they come from? Jake-man's book, The Divided Skies explained where the Tuskegee Airman came from. It gives an in-depth description of the inception of the Tuskegee Institute and its formation, which ultimately gave birth to the Tuskegee Airmen. After their superb flight training, a select few made a major impact in the war through their excellent pilot skills. They earned the reputation as the Tuskegee Airmen.

In March 1942, at the Tuskegee Army Air Field, in Alabama, five men received the silver wings of Army Air Forces pilots: George S. Roberts, Benjamin: O. Davis, Jr., Charles H. Be Bow, Jr., Mac Ross, and Lemuel R. Custis: these men completed standard, army-flight classroom instructions.

Before these five men entered the program, black men could not serve in the military! Obviously, racial exclusion in the Navy continued on many years after the first black men graduated from Tuskegee Institute. However, that did not thwart their God given ability to beat the odds and rise above the circumstances to rise to the acme of their goal.

The events of September 11 has reiterated my previous statements. That each of us, at some point in our lives, has experienced the consequences of rejection in one way or the other: like the Mosaic Nucleus of the Human Race, rejected by the hideous act of those hijackers.

In conclusion of this chapter, let us not forget the Acmatic achievements and contributions of Secretary of State Colin Powell and White House National Security Advisor Condoleezza Rice… And who can forget the redoubtable Oprah Winfrey, Queen of the talk shows! The biggest star-maker the literary world had ever seen, who personally contributed to the most successful time for the publishing world through the nascence of OPRAH'S Book Club; and the invaluable contribution of national and international literary out-reach to the world of literacy.

Armed with the knowledge that we have the potentials to be all that we can be: not tacit, but vocal, with a sense of purpose, you owe it to yourself and us to be an assiduous member of society.

If the intransigent Rosa Park had not been resolute in her refusal to accede to the unjust demand of those who insisted she give up her inalienable right, and sit at the available seat where she was relegated to sit at the back of the bus, on December 1, 1955, perhaps we would be reading a different chapter in the history of the civil rights movement.

The evidence shows that, despite the plethora of rejections, and the vicissitudes of daily life, with much fortitude and a considerable amount of mental gymnastics, any individual can break out of their creative chrysalis and achieve the recognition they deserve. Further information is Available in my third book titled: *ROMW vs. RAMB [Acronym] Read Only My Word vs. Random Access Make Believe.*

CHAPTER 6

A Winner Never Quits and a Quitter Never Wins

A winner never quits and a quitter never wins; is a statement of fact that will stand the test of time! This truism is evident throughout the history of the human race… most notable in the 1955 incident that enriched us all, the intransient courage of the respectable Rosa Park.

If she had not been resolute in her stand against discrimination and rejection, the people of color would still be relegated to the back of the bus, and the end of lines, until a person of more combative and unabashed personality came along: resulting in the implementation of inevitable change in this country and the world at large.

The inexorable zeal of those courageous pioneers was not a peripatetic exercise in futility, but an exercise in true altruism. Had she and other brave civil rights leaders like Dr. King and others had quit amid the flagitious rule of the segregated elites of that era, the minority communities of the world would not have benefited from the legacy of their struggle.

The record shows the intransient activists of the civil rights movements of the 50s and 60s did not obsequiously accede to the imperative command of the repressive rule of that era!

OK! Much notoriety has been given to the famous personalities and pioneers of history. Let us talk about the not so famous individuals throughout history and in our time. You and I, whose names are not household words.

Everyone has a story to tell in their own words, even though it may not make the newspaper headlines; or prime time-news. Nevertheless, we all have our own encounter with life's quotidian struggle of one form or the other.

Trials and errors

Let us use a carpenter for example... He decides to lay the framework for a building project. He estimated the cost of the project and, due to his miscalculations came up short of money and materials in the middle of the project.

The question is: should he quit the project because of his error in judgment and negligence? No! He should assess the situation resulting from his error, make the necessary corrections and continue with the project, or come to some compensatory settlement of the cost incurred and not let it impair his ability to start his next project.

Likewise, a plumber would not quit his job just because he made a mistake by breaking a water main during the course of his work. He should not dwell on his mistake, but learn from it, by making sure it does not recur.

One should think of the many successes in one's career, before a particular mistake, and not let this mistake cause you to ruminate on the thought of quitting. In each situation, you should just think of the good days, learn from the mistakes of the past, and move on with your life.

A mechanic never quits because of his mistakes

A mechanic never quits his job because he installed a brake system the wrong way, in light of the potential disastrous consequence of that big mistake. The solution is the same as previously stated. He should correct the problem and assume the responsibility for the cost incurred: he should learn from his mistake and not quit.

A technician does not quit his job because he installed the wrong parts in a piece of electronic equipment; neither should he dwell on the mistake but learn from it and go on doing what he can do best and not ruminate on the mistake indefinitely.

You do not have to be a psychiatrist or psychologist to speak on this issue. Anyone who has experienced the vicissitudes of daily life can concur with theses stated facts.

Whenever you and I are faced with an unfair situation in life, let us be inspired by those who have faced similar situations before and face the challenge head on and not quit, just because the situation seems insurmountable.

For example, your entire career has been one success after another. Recently you maladroitly made a mess of an important project. You became so embarrassed in front of your coworkers that you now hate going to work.

As stated previously, the solution is to eschew the negative impulse to laden yourself with guilt that will further impair your ability to focus on your previous successes! Learn from your mistakes and move forward.

No one has a monopoly on failures! The expert will tell you how many people write and complain about their failures as if their failures are unique. With all due respect, your failures are not unique, despite its ineffable description. You and I, as members of the human race, are not immune from failures! Therefore, you are not alone in this struggle.

In my books titled: ***A Myopic Life Resonated*** and the book: ***Romw vs. Ramb [Acronym] Read Only My Word vs. Random Access Make Believe,*** I have written extensively on the cause and effect of failures and cures for such ubiquity among us.

The redoubtable Albert Einstein is a paradigmatic example among many other intellectual geniuses who have had their experiences of failures, yet these Acmatic achievement have inspired us all.

Mistakes are common among us but; is not a recipe for doing wrong; therefore, we must always strive to do right and not wrong! The consequence of mistakes is always costly.

Making a big deal out of failure

Arguably, some people think you learn from your mistakes, yet others believe failure builds character. This statement may surprise some people: nevertheless, do you think people who focus on their successes rather than on their failures can be more confident and more successful than people who don't?

You will learn more when you are not too egotistical about your mistakes! People learn more from their failures than from not trying. It has been said, "You learn more when you cry than when you smile."

Both success and failure build character

The question is not if failure builds character or not, the important thing is not to make a big deal of it. Yes, many people fail; nonetheless, some are more resilient to failure than others are. These people do not think failure is important. They learn more from their success. Do you think these people are happier and less stressed because of what their attitudes may be like? If they are less stressed, they will probably be more successful in life. What is your opinion?

I think it is safe to assume that the hundreds of heroic fire fighters and police officers who at the World Trade Center in their normal duty, did not think their effort was an act in futility: when they did not save everyone from those towering infernos on September 11, or from any other burning building where the lives of civilians, fire fighters or police officers were lost.

Although hundreds of those heroic fire fighters and polices officers never made it out of that horrific disaster alive, their meritorious act of true altruism demonstrated they were not failures. They did not escape the towering infernos themselves. Nevertheless, the Alacrity of their response to the call of duty, and the hundred of lives saved, made their effort a tremendous success.

The question asked: Suppose you had to learn an intricate task on your job. Would you rather learn from someone who had always done it right? Alternatively, would you rather learn from someone who has learned from experience about the pitfalls and unforeseen challenges?

What is your opinion? Alternatively, would you rather learn from the maxim, Hard knocks often make the best teacher? On the other hand, it is a natural tendency of human nature to always gravitate to a winner.

You must be prepared to take on the nuances of life with fortitude and eschew those problematic pitfalls with celerity.

The myriad occupational hazards and mistakes are too numerous to mention; nonetheless, these few examples illustrate the point and the truism that a winner never quits and a quitter never wins.

CHAPTER 7

How to Deal with Failure: Not as the Pessimist Who Sees the Glass Half Empty, but an Optimist Who Sees it Half Full, Not at Its Nadir.

An epigraph by William B. Sprague ...
"Do not wait to strike till the iron is hot; but make it hot by striking."

How to deal with failure may be of interest to anyone who is experiencing it at any given time. In the interim of such hackneyed occurrences in one's life, there is a sense of hopelessness that permeates the heart and soul of that person who is grappling with that ephemeral situation.

If a person loses, his job or experiences any of the varieties of life's challenges, in light of what happened on September 11, some may be resilient enough to make a com- back, by picking up the broken pieces of his or her life and trying something new.

Others may not be so resilient, and fall through the cracks and crannies of life; where there were no safety nets to break the fall: Therefore, that unfortunate person may resort to begging.

FISH STORY

"BROTHER, CAN YOU SPARE A DIME?"

"Brother, Can You Spare a Dime?"

There was a stereotypical expression in our society that coined the phrase "Brother, can you spare a dime?" This reminds me of a situation, while I was walking down the street of the Bronx, N.Y. I saw a homeless man walking the streets, searching the garbage cans, looking for food. I offered him some loose change I had in my pocket.

The man refused to accept my offer. That is a classic example of an ungrateful person! The solution to this segment of our society however, is charity with the incentive to help oneself. Allow me at this time to recommend this plan of action that suggests the following:

"Give a man a fish, and he will feed himself for a day! Teach him how to fish, and he will feed himself and his family for the rest of his life!"

With that sound advice, a person has the option of pursuing his dreams from the viewpoint of the optimist, who sees the glass "half full," not as the pessimist who sees it half empty, or at its nadir!

Pardon me of this slight digression as it relates to another subject!

Help is on the way

Help is on the way! A theme echoed during the Presidential Election Campaign of 2000: The debate was about beefing up the allegedly fledging U.S. Armed Forces.

Although one of the major issues of the campaign was on Foreign Policy, nevertheless, domestic agendas were hotly debated. Among the issues debated was how to meet the needs of society's poor and indigent citizens.

As I suggested previously: One way to deal with this segment of society is to teach a man how to fish (literally or figuratively)... In addition, he will be able to feed his family for the rest of his life.

Teach the unskilled person a trade; provide a safety net when possible to individuals who can't pull themselves up by their bootstraps. Provide spiritual and moral support so they can help themselves and others along the way up the ladder of success and upward mobility.

Many people have forgotten their roots! As soon as they have climbed the ladder of success, they quickly forget those at the lower echelon of society.

This not only applies to secular members of society, but even to those of the clergy. Unfortunately, there are many who came from a humble nascence, have reached the acme of their stewardship, and now have forgotten some who are not members of the local body.

I am thankful for my accomplishments. I also contribute to the poor consistently. There was a time in my life when I was in need of the basic essentials of life, though, not to the extent described in my first book!

Today, I consider myself blessed, being able to finance my four books without support, morally or spiritually; especially from those who have within their power to help promulgate the auspicious message I have to convey.

Name recognition vs. lifetime reward

Most aspiring writers know that writing is not just for the purpose of making wads of money, but for the sense of satisfaction and accomplishment; knowing that when the finished product is in the hands of the reading public it can be a fulfilling reward, knowing that you have made a difference, by helping someone through the written word.

To the aspiring first-time writer: Don't be discouraged if you fail in your first attempt to have your book published. Surveys show that many of today's best-selling authors have had their manuscript rejected numerous times before it was accepted and finally published.

One author had his manuscript rejected numerous times before it was accepted, and it became a best seller. The world will not stop, despite our failures. In the majority of situations there is always a remedy. Some people have an extraordinary resilient escape mechanism, not allowing themselves to be victims of circumstances and are considered examples of survival of the fittest.

Most failures are learning experiences that build character and reinforce our efforts to focus on the things we do best and are likely to succeed at.

We should not let our failures become such an irritant to the extent of letting them continue to cause a deleterious effect on our emotional well being, like a perpetual burr under a jockey's saddle.

The winning idea...

Let us stay focused on the winning idea, the things that matter most. Those things that can make a difference in our life and the lives of others ...

Simple things like a kind gesture, a simple thank you to someone who has been kind to you; or even mean to you, for that matter. An acknowledgement of receipt from an unimportant person who has presented you with a gift, no matter how insignificant the gift may be. What seems meretricious to you may pass as salient beauty, loveliness, and attractiveness to another.

Failure to reciprocate with kindness, may lead to a feeling of rejection that can have a deleterious effect on someone's self-esteem. You must avoid this with celerity.

CHAPTER 8

The Thrill of Victory and the Agony of Defeat…

Every individual knows how it feels to experience the thrill of victory and the agony of defeat … the accolades given to the stalwart Albert Einstein, whose theory of relativity most historian's claim was an Acmatic breakthrough in the discovery of science and mathematics.

Despite his breathtaking achievement, however, his life was not without trials and errors. He experienced many failures before he rose to the acme of his achievements.

Every successful scientist and inventor can speak volumes of their failure, due to trials and errors during the course of their experiments, before they succeeded in ending previous unsuccessful attempts to break out of their creative chrysalis, and achieve recognition for their invention.

One can safely assume that it must have caused many sleepless nights as they tirelessly burned the midnight oil: as they endeavored to succeed in their experiments. Just imagine how many trials and errors they experienced before they arrived at the correct formula.

A person does not have to be a scientist, or a member of the esoteric group of scientists and engineers, to concur that in order to succeed in this transient world, you have to be resilient and not be a jejune quitter, when you experienced failure and disappointments in the vicissitudes of daily life.

Let us take a second look at some of the many "rags to riches" "thrill of victory! And the agony of defeat stories."

The average men and women on the street who became rich and famous movie stars, recording artists, boxers, baseball super stars, etc., all theses individuals have experienced the thrill of victory, from been an ordinary person to the kind of contributing member of society they became.

In the sphere of this transient life, you too can be all that you want to be as long as you and I keep things in perspective.

An old adage articulates the following quote:

"... If you want to jump over a fence and you aim for the treetop, you may not clear the fence... If you aim for the moon, however, in all probability you are bound to clear the fence."

The above allegory may have some semblance of truth in its descriptive analysis, depending on how laterally we interpret it. Nevertheless, we can adhere to the practical aspect of it.

The moral of the story is this: Any able-bodied individual can make it in this great country if given a fair chance, with a level playing field.

In all fairness, we know there is a myriad hurdles to cross over on the way to success. You and I can make it if we try hard enough, be persistent about it and not be a diffident quitter amid our relentless pursuit of our goals and assiduous aspirations.

Since a couple of decades ago, we have seen a large number of small businesses and young entrepreneurs emerge from obscurity into large corporations, and even make it in the ranks of the Fortune Five Hundred.

The Internet, for example, has produced many multimillionaires. Many started as home based-businesses from their basement and garages, kitchen tables, and some, even from their bedrooms.

Most of these individuals, who have made it from rags to riches into the corporate world, have had their share of failures during the course of their efforts to succeed. Each has their own story to tell of their upward-mobility struggle up the ladder of success and how they overcame failures and defeats along the way.

This parvenu is evident in the game of sports... In heavyweight championship fights, and all sports: Think of how humiliating it can be to boxing champions who go down on the canvas from a devastating knockout punch, the ultimate agony of defeat.

On the other hand, imagine the euphoric feeling of ineffable expression after a champ knocks-out his opponent cold. The thrill of victory: and the agony of defeat for the looser.

The continuing saga of "the thrill of victory!" "And the agony of defeat."

Baseball: America's Favorite Pastime

Most people who are baseball fans, have experienced the rush of adrenaline that flows in the brain during an All Star, and World Series game, or any game clincher, for that matter.

A loaded-bases two-outs-in-the-ninth inning game can be an arduous task, as a reliever needs to get his last strike out. If he blew the save, by giving up the game- winning homer; or a base hit with the winning run for the opposing team, it is all over for the losing team. That would be an agony of defeat. On the other hand: the winning team would celebrate the thrill of victory, bruited by the media.

This is indicative of all sports and the vicissitude game of daily life. The good news is: this too will pass! The apparent defeat is short-lived.

"While the earth remains," there will always be a next season in the game of sports, and the way of life. However, this assurance is for those who are determined not to be a jejune quitter in the game of life when the going gets rough, or in the heat of battle.

A paragon example is a Biblical story of the leader of the children of Israel, as he chose twenty and two thousand men to fight against his enemies, but was told by the captain of the Army of the Lord to first put the men to a test, to prove their fitness for battle against their enemies.

After the initial test of several thousand men, only 300 were chosen and found fit for battle against their enemies. The others were sent home.

This is a classic example of the winning walk with the giver of life, like those who become winners, and not quitters. Nevertheless, those who failed the test to be a good soldier; were sent home... They perhaps picked up their armors and moved on to their respected places in society; doing the things they are capable of doing.

For more information on the principles and applications of "The Thrill of Victory and the Agony of Defeat," ***read the books, A Myopic Life Resonated: and, Romw vs. Ramb by Simeon Johnson***

As stated previously: The average person has a tendency to quit after a few failed attempts at something... not so with Albert Einstein! His many failed experiments did not thwart his creative ability and his resiliency to be all that he could be, to become one of the world's greatest scientists of the twentieth century.

The assiduousness of the stalwart Albert Einstein reiterates the premise of this chapter's title: The thrill of victory! And the agony of defeat ... On the other hand, a winner never quits, and a quitter never wins!

CHAPTER 9

TECHNOLOGY ON THE CUTTING EDGE

Every generation since the Industrial Revolution has had nostalgia for the simpler times of their generation…

We are living in the age of rapid growth in science and engineering to the point of what we now experience as information overload. Approximately every eighteen months there is a new introduction of consumer products vis-à-vis electronics gadgets etc.

Many people, especially senior citizens, complain that, as soon as they become acquainted with a new electronic product, along came an upgraded version of sorts, which in many cases are more complicated to work with. The vocabulary used in today's electronic vernacular is astounding to the average consumer.

Baby Boomers

Among the most populace generation in American history is the Baby Boomers, which made its entrance onto the earth's stage in the 50s. During the Boomers first decade, a myriad of new words have entered the vernacular of America's vocabulary.

The Industrial Revolution has given us a quantum leap into the age of innovative technology. Along with the introduction of cutting-edge technology is the vernacular of the Baby Boomers, Words like fiber optic, CAT Scan, HTML, home page URL, MPEG-3, desktop publishing, DVD, junk mail, carbon dating, OSD, H-bomb, panic button, Set top box, world class, TV/VCR Combos, and many others'.

As the Boomers became an adult, and broke out of her creative chrysalis and become of age, and ultimately, an empty-nester, and soon acquired many new words numbering in the thousands annually; after turning on the spotlight to make a reality check of her newly found treasure.

As she finds these effervescent material treasures, she soon realizes, from the diurnal experience of life and its challenges that it introduce, the stressed out syndrome from the fast track spent networking with yuppies, etc.

It is not surprising why the Boomers began feeling stressed out and overworked in many ways.

As the "me" generation grew from its early beginning into a senescent disoriented Boomer. They found the corporate business ventures of American society appear to be capitalist oriented, so the efforts of business was to devise a lexicon of new terms to describe the realities of new venture capital.

The 1980s and 90s were said to be the golden age of venture capital, golden parachutes, golden hand-shakers. Technology, in partnership with business, also gave us ATMs, bank cards, debit cards, terms like domestic partners, glass ceiling, max out, Pin, power breakfast, power lunches, Telemarketing, entry-level white knights etc.,

Word Phrase

Boomers were inundated with a myriad of technological terms that made their entry into technical dictionary, words like call waiting, bullet train, (HDTV) Highdefnition TV, Set-top box, cable-ready, MTV, (ISDN) Multimedia, PDF Files, GPG Files, and many other word usages and terminology.

Included in the terminology are the medical terms such as DNA, attributing to the most recent advance and breathtaking potential of stem cell research and human cloning.

CHAPTER 10

Technological Advance at Its Zenith

We are in awe at the technological advance of our time! The events of the day are a paradigm example of the advances of innovative technology, and the pros and cons of its effect here in the U.S. and the world...

The insidious act of either foreign or domestic terrorism that is wreaking havoc in the U.S. and the global communities with Anthrax is the act of a stoic evil person, acquiring knowledge, not for the greater good, but for his diabolical purpose.

The descriptive analysis of the foregoing chapter, has given us an in-depth overview of the past few decades and its effect on our generation. There should be no doubt that the futuristic forecast, thousands of years ago by the Prophet Daniel, is evident today.

The emergence of the Industrial Revolution has seen that the results of those predictions of almost three thousand years ago, are without question, the evidence that we are living in the last days of Daniel's prophetic forecast that knowledge shall increase in the last days. Who can argue with that? We have come a long way since the days of chariots and horses in light of today's events, have we not?

Chariots and horses were the fastest means of transportation in ancient times compared to the events of September 11, 2001. The comparison is like night and day, not to mention all the modern inventions of the 21st Century, by the evidence of what we are witnessing today.

Railroad

The railways of the 16th Century, for example, includes a single rail pulled by horses along wooden rails, used for mining purposes. The modern railroad began with the steam locomotive pioneered by the Englishmen, Richard Trevithick and George Stephenson in the early 1800s.

The Japanese delivered high-speed passenger trains, such as the Bullet and TGv trains. France and Germany also experimented with magnet levitation trains on short tracks in several countries.

Automobiles

The late Henry Ford, an American industrialist, pioneered the manufacturing of the first Model T cars while working as a machinist and engineer with the Edison Co. in his spare time. in 1892 and in 1903, he organized the Ford Motor Co. and designed and built the Model T, with over 15 million cars sold, before the model was discontinued in 1928 to make way for a new design of the Model A to meet the growing competition.

In reality, the men and women who played a pivotal role in the fulfillment of the technological breakthrough by the inspirational prediction of the Prophet Daniel should be cognizant that those pioneers were not quitters, when things weren't going their way.

They resisted the stigmas of failure, persisted in their lucubratory effort, by burning the midnight oil to pursue their dreams, and became winners.

In the old days, the Creator has always used able men and women to fulfill His intended purpose. Like always, and in the future, He will use whom He will, to carry out His purpose.

The Airplane

On December 17, 1903, Americans Orville and Wilbur Wright flew the first airplane near Kitty Hawk, N.C.

Daniel's experiences with his futuristic predictions were divinely inspired. Yet, in his mortal state of mind he was overwhelmed and fainted. Not surprising considering the proliferation and development of the technological advances of our time.

Hardly anyone who witnessed the breathtaking Space Shuttle and other space Crafts from Cape Canaveral and other launching pads; are not in awe at the sonic boom during the blast-off of those crafts into outer space. Daniel, however, was a man of like passion as we are." He was no less awestruck by what he envisioned for the future.

After Daniel's fainting episode, the revelator strengthened him and told him his vision was not for his time, but of the end time. With that said, we should be cognizant of the signs of the time! We are living in the last days of Daniel's prediction.

Pivotal devices that paved the way for the Information Age...

Le DeForest ushered in the beginning of the information technological revolution in 1915, which paved the way for the high technology breakthrough of the information age.

Before that time, however, the performance of telephone network, were constrained by electromagnetic devices. Nationwide, the practicality of telephone calls was almost prohibitive.

Broadcast radio and TV signals were almost impossible to fundamentally realize without the aid of the electronic amplifier and oscillator to facilitate its use.

The vacuum tube had an immediate effect on the long-lines telephone network and saw the establishment of radio services the late 1919. This was only eclipsed in 1956 by TAT1, the first Trans-Atlantic telephone cable with an initial 36 simultaneous speech circuits.

The cost of the services was prohibitive for the average citizen. By 1986, there were seven U.K. –to- U.S.A. cables with a total of 1200 speech circuits, and six satellites providing 57,000 circuits.

At the time, TAT8 was installed… The technology had moved unto fiber optics with 7,680 base circuits in one cable. Today's systems designed with capacities 1, 000 fold the capacity of TAT8 and five million fold that TAT1.

Transistor Revolution

The transistor revolution emerges as an essential component of integrated circuits: It is used in almost every application of our lives, since its discovery by the American physicists John Braden, Walter H. Bratten, and William Schockley in 1948.

Almost 3,000 years after the Prophet Daniel predicted technology in the futuristic increase of knowledge, we are witnessing the result of the benefits, pros, and cons, of those heart patients whose lives are greatly improved by the intricate devices in their bodies as a result of the increase of knowledge.

The partially blind person in some cases is able to see, with modern technological procedures. Many who could not see are now able to see.

Robotic operations are now conducted from a considerable distance by remote control, without a significant loss of blood. Time does not permit me to list all the benefits of today's technology and its applications in our lives.

All the above-mentioned are a direct byproduct of the vacuum tube technology, how it has revolutionized our way of life in many ways.

Integrated Circuit

The integrated circuits (IC) are the direct byproducts of the vacuum tube and transistor technology that are used as computer memory circuits and microprocessors. All are byproduct of the vacuum tube technology.

The Age of Miniaturization

The age of miniaturization and innovative technology, brought about by the invention of the vacuum tube technology, is far different in size, compared to the enormous size of the first prototype computer built by the military, occupying space the size of a large room compared to today's miniature hand-held Palm Pilot etc.

Blue-Tooth Technology

As the cutting edge of high technology advances, along comes the Blue-tooth technology. The potential of this technology is enormous.

Here is a quote from a document at the Motorola Blue-tooth website at www.mot.com/bluetooth: "Blue tooth in its most basic form is cable replacement. Where cable now connects many devices, a wireless Blue tooth connection will provide low cost wireless communications and networking between PC, mobile phones, and other devices"

This will enable untethered, wireless connectivity to the Internet and other devices, anytime, anywhere. Blue tooth based on a global radio frequency (RF) Standard, which operates on the 2.4 GHZ ISM band, providing license-free operation in the United States, most of Europe and Japan.

The fact that companies numbering in the thousands, from cell-phone manufactures, and manufacturers of IC chips that will provide the connectivity have joined a Blue- tooth special interest group (SIG), implies that this will soon be a major technology.

Nine well-known companies in the Blue-tooth SIG constitute a "Promoter Group" tending the development of the technology: 3Com, Erickson, Intel, IBM, Lucent, Microsoft, Motorola, Nokia and Toshiba.

Blue-tooth has evolved from basic cellular digital radio designs implemented in mobile phones since the early 1980s. It will enable users to connect a wide range of computing and telecommunications devices easily and quickly without the need for cables. It will expand communications capabilities for computers, mobile phones and other mobile devices in the office and outside the office.

Here is a little technical information about Blue- tooth. First, communication should be fast. The raw data rate of the technology can be as high as 1Mbps, certainly a lot faster than communications with a 56kbs model. A device with Blue tooth capability will be able to exchange information within about a 30-foot radius.

As to the cost, Motorola says that when the adoption of the technology is widespread, and manufacturing economies attained, the cost of providing devices with Blue- tooth technology should not be significant.

If you are concerned that someone else might gain access to your data via the Blue-tooth connections that is unlikely to happen. The technology is designed to be secure under most normal conditions. To be specific, the Blue-tooth specifications include the following features: data encryption, low-layer support for user authentication, fast- frequency hopping (1600 hops per second), output power control that automatically limits power to optimally fit the distance between connected device.

Again, according to Motorola, "these features provide both layer physical radio security that is unlikely to be eavesdropped on.

As well as a mechanism to support, higher layers of security such as pass words and Pin's like all communication technologies, there is some level of risk of exposure to unintended parties, but Bluetooth wireless technology is designed to make that very unlikely and difficult to do."

Things That Blue Tooth Can Do

The things Blue tooth will do for people are truly amazing. For example, use of the technology will have instant, automatic, access to business and personal data. All of the Blue tooth devices will have access to e-mail and the Internet from anywhere.

A person with one of these units will be able to network with airlines, hotels, theaters, retail stores and restaurants.

The Motorola web site mentioned earlier includes several pages of slides that show some of the things that will be possible. For example, one slide has this scenario: "While in a meeting, you access your PDA (personal digital assistant) to send your presentation to the electronic whiteboard."

"You record meeting minutes on your PDA and wirelessly transfer these minutes to the attendees before they leave the meeting."

Alternatively, how about this picture: "You arrived at the airport. A long line formed for ticketing and seat assignment. You avoid the line, using your PDA to present an electronic ticket, and automatically select your seat. The airline's on line system checker identification via the "ID- tag" feature built into your PDA and confirms your reserved seat."

The slide set includes a number of other situations in which their technology can make the lives of people easier.

Continuing with the way it can help on a trip: The presentation mentions simplification of the process of renting a car, and checking into a hotel.

Most likely you have seen the commercial: a person, presumably in Italy, is talking on his cell phone; he eyes a soft-drink machine. He is thirsty. He reaches in his pocket. No change. He sees many coins in a fountain, reaches in. A nun standing by gives him a disapproving look. He looks guilty. Then a young woman comes by, stands in front of the soft-drink machine, punches a few numbers into her PDA (or cell phone) and out pops a can of soda. She takes a big gulp. No doubt this is an application of Blue-tooth technology. Pretty slick...

In addition, what happens if you lose your PDA and someone picks it up? If you have never had a password on your computer at work or at home, you better be sure your Blue-tooth enabled PDA is password protected. In addition, do not forget the password.

While Blue-tooth will make life easer much of the time, can you see it leading to some spectacular mess? What happens if you're in that meeting ready to transfer that presentation to the electronic whiteboard and your batteries give out, or some other malfunction occurs to your PDA?

This technology is so new that we are not sure what the implication might be for the consumer service. However, we feel this is a technology that every technician needs to know. As the Blue-tooth devices proliferate, and the mist begins to clear, we will provide continuing coverage of this breathtaking technology.

"The fact that companies numbering in the thousands...have joined a Blue tooth special interest group (SIG) implies that this will soon be a major technology." Editor Nils Conrad Persson ES&T Magazine

All these breathtaking new inventions since the Industrial Revolution have set the pace for rapid acceleration and growth of the technological age in the industrial world.

The world at large is the recipient and beneficiary of these developments, a truly remarkable accomplishment of human kind. Further information on the pros and cons of today's technology regarding Daniel's prediction are written in my book ***Romw vs. Ramb.***

Comment

With the emergence of the Baby Boomers, the acceleration of innovative technology has inspired the pioneers of the new frontiers to break new grounds into the future with Celerity.

In addition to the developments of modern inventions, it produced a plethora of unknown potentials, and a paucity of humility.

CHAPTER 11

STEM CELL RESEARCH AND HUMAN CLONING

Stem cell research, human and animal cloning! Is this a subject to ignore? What is your opinion?

Although the following discussion is an impalpable biological and scientific science known only to the esoteric minds, the resultant moral and ethical implications are not esoteric by any stretch of the imagination.

The issues of this thought-provoking subject and new scientific breakthrough, is ineffable from a nonprofessional's point of view. I will elaborate on the subject, not from a doctiloquent point of view, but from my perspective as a concerned citizen endeavoring to heighten awareness of this unknown subject with a perspective enlistment.

Q & A

The following Q & A is a colloquial discussion by two experts on the pros and cons on the subject of cloning.

"…The issue of cloning burst onto the world consciousness in 1997 when Scottish scientists announced they had cloned a sheep named Dolly. Since then, goats, pigs, mice, and cows also cloned." In addition, many scientists expect to clone a human in the world within a year. "… The technique to cloning a human would be to remove the nuclei of a woman's egg and replace them with the nucleus from any cell from any part of a body, male or female, and the resulting embryo used for medical research. "Therapeutic cloning, with the hope of some day healing people by replacing their diseased cells, or the embryo could be implanted into a woman's womb and allowed to be developed into a baby reproductive cloning. The baby would be genetically identical to the donor of the cell nucleus."

Both types of cloning are widely opposed, but cloning for medical research has more support than cloning for reproduction.

"… Recently France and Germany asked the United Nations to approve a ban on all reproductive cloning worldwide. At the time of this writing, the United States prohibits reproductive cloning, but there is no federal law against either kind of cloning,"

The experts state their opposition to reproductive cloning by saying… "Reproductive cloning is something, which has the whole world throwing up their hands in horror."

"…The notion that you make human beings, basically by photocopying them, rather by the process of procreation through love. You can photocopy what you want; you can pick the person you want to copy; but this is appalling. It is a wakeup call as we discover what the new biotechnology holds in store for us."

(Q) There is also the problem of learning to do it, isn't their? In the creation there are many defective and deformed creatures.

(A) "Well, the evidence is, this is an experimental technique which is highly ineffective."

"At a recent congruence in Washington, where some scientists said they are to give the go-ahead and clone a baby, everybody was horrified, partly because it was said: "Well, you want to try dozens, and dozens of times before you get a normal one." 'This is experimenting on young human beings!' "

(Q) Should the decision on that be up to the adult person? Shouldn't each adult, male or female, have the right to decide what happens to its genetic material?"

(A) "I think that's an appalling suggestion!" "All children are people!" "They are other people!" "They certainly shouldn't be things we make, because we chose!' "

One of the participating professors states his position, pros and cons against cloning. He states that there are two arguments that are generally given. One: "People are to have access to any medically safe technology to have the sort of child they want to have. This falls, so the argument goes, under the sphere of privacy and reproductive liberty. Keep the Government out of our bedroom! That sort of rhetoric we all are familiar with."

"The other argument is to say! Look, there may be some scenario in which the compassionate among us would say, go ahead: For instance, imagine a woman involved in a traffic accident, and she lost a fetus late term in her pregnancy, and she also lost the capacity ever to conceive again! Would you allow her to clone what is lost in order to somehow continue that pregnancy?"

"Or some people would say, look! There are some families, which are inevitably cutoff, maybe for one survivor, cut off by the holocaust! Would you allow that one survivor to be cloned as a way of bringing technology in, to allow sort of a final vindication over the Nazis?"

One of the opposing professors inveighs strongly against the idea of cloning. He argues that those posing arguments… if you want to defeat Hitler or the Nazis, you do it by opposing anti-Semitism and racism, when we experience a lost cause for griefs. Not for some high-tech concern."

He also stated that there are other arguments, more substantial, that cloning would confuse relationships. What is cloning? Is it a twin? Is it a child? "I don't know if anybody would know how to rear a clone properly. I think there are substantial reasons not to clone." I am open to carry on the debate. But for right now, my vote is against reproductive cloning! "

(Q) The host asked one of the professors: Let me turn now to therapeutic cloning, as you have said, so-called therapeutic cloning for medical research to cure disease. What is wrong with doing that?

(A) "Some of the disturbing things about the present debate is that people seem to be thinking, by saying, this may cure terrible diseases, and we said you could do it. We had a thing written called the Nuremberg code, after the Second World War that said, You do not experiment on human beings! Not to mention tiny human beings... In addition, you certainly do not have to take the pro-life views to take the view that the early human embryo needs protection from this kind of experimental work."

(Q) So your point is that early embryos would have to be destroyed in the process, despite the status of the fetus?

(A) "... Well, plainly! The early embryo is a human being, a member of our species, and whether or not we take the view, for example, whenever you take on abortion, there is a wide concern that we should not experiment on tiny human beings, or indeed deliberately create them for experiments."

Six years ago the Washington Post, which is hardly a conservative journal, said, "It would be unconscionable to create embryos just to destroy them through experiments and many people of pro choice would agree with that point of view, that this is something we should never do."

(Q) Professor: What is your argument on that?

(A) "... Well, I think it is permissible! However, it must be under the most rigorous regulatory environment. I think, as a precious commodity, that there should be an active Federal role."

"But personally, I believe they are not yet of the status, morally speaking of a human being! They don't rise to the level of falling under the protection of the Nuremberg Code."

(Q) Do you think if permitted for medical research, that a cloned embryo is preventable from use in reproduction?

(A) "Well I think if we have the proper Federal concourse-and-regularity environment we can say very clearly, a limited number of embryos, ever to be created by cloning, or other means for research purposes and, research only through 14 days, and at the end of that, 'Who in their right mind would have implanted such an embryo that had been subject to scientific research? You don't know what kind of terrible consequence that might bring in the world.' "

Conclusion:

"Well, there are a lot of people out there who certainly aren't in their right mind! In addition, we do live in a world, in which, in this country: we have the most liberal regime, with almost no control at all of any country in the west. Secondly… if we are ever going to start cloning, even reproductive cloning; is to get Congress to legislate laws, pros-and-con about cloning,"

Comments:

With the plethora of information provided by the experts in the colloquial discussion that preceded … the moral of the discussion in question is this:

If history has taught us anything, we should learn from the mistakes of the past and recent events.

A classic example is the authentic story of the tree of knowledge, of good and evil, described in the genesis of creation, a temptation, our first parents could not resist. They acceded to the suggestion of the deceiver that if they eat of the tree of knowledge, of good and evil, they would become like gods.

The result is what we are witnessing today! Men's desire to break out of his creative chrysalis to achieve the recognition he thinks he deserves.

Erudite Man's Desire for Change

Man's mordant wit and erudite desire to change the status quo of, the established social order has been a pervasive social dilemma since the beginning of time.

Some changes are for the greater good that benefits humankind, while others lead to the detriment of society. Case in point: With the nascence of the Industrial Revolution, compared to today's innovative technological age, we are witnessing the enormous effect of change on society. One does not have to look far to see the effect of such change.

The industrial world has influenced our lives in many ways... Its innovative change has transformed our lives for better or for worse! In light of recent events, we have seen some of its worst and best byproducts at work.

The idea that stem cell research and cloning will result in a panacea cure for all is an illusive path into the unknown. No one knows for sure where this relatively new and breathtaking technology will lead.

Just think of a person born from a clone experiment: Have these scientists ruminated on the spiritual and moral aspects of the dilemma this individual will face as to who his Creator is?

It is understandably normal to assume that the unbelieving scientists have not given this idea second thought. Nevertheless, the relevancy of the subject matter is of paramount concern

The Scripture spoke of similar concerns that are tantamount to the subject in question, when a certain man came to the One who holds the original patent of the creation of man and woman, and asked Him about life after death.

There was a question asked. "If seven brethren having claims to one wife at the resurrection, whose wife shall she be?" Do you see the relevant concern of the subject matter?

In the process of cloning there will inevitably be some selections and rejections of unwanted cells or embryos. What will happen to the souls of these rejected embryos during these experiments?

Will they appear before the real Creator as not having an eternal soul? Will these questions be like those seven husbands having the same wife? (Mark 12:19-23). The rejected- embryos question as to who is their creator.

These and other probing questions need to be addressed regarding the ineffable consequences of cloning before we proceed precipitously with this newly discovered innovative technology, of stem sell research of animal and human cloning.

The decision of scientists to go full-speed ahead is a cursory decision not methodically thought out as stated before. The consequence of change has its pros and cons. Therefore, it is for this reason we should embrace the positive aspect of change with Alacrity and eschew its negative application with Celerity.

CHAPTER 12

In This Time of Universal Grief

In this time of universal grief, what the world needs now is the perfect blood transfusion that can heal soul, body and spirit. In light of September 11, and the events of the day, my book ***A Myopic Life Resonate***d describes the perfect formula for such a time as this. Read all about a father's venomous hatred for his daughter's changed life! Jovial witty, funny! A Bold act to eschew and not repeated. A must read...

Although America and the world communities mourn the loss of hundreds of New York's Bravest firefighters, police officers, and thousands of men, women and children on September 11, a day that will live in infamy, the greatest terrorist act perpetrated on America in the history of this country, the hideous act of those stoic evildoers has not destroyed our spirit of love for the rest of our fellow man.

Therefore, we respectfully mourn the loss resulting from the enormity of the hideous act of terrorism perpetrated on America, including the ever-increasing threat of anthrax that is causing terror in this country. Nevertheless, let us not forget the other deadly diseases that are plaguing our communities and the world at large.

AIDS

AIDS is a subject society cannot afford to ignore! Statistically, the alarming number of people dying annually from AIDS worldwide according to estimates from the Joint United Nations Program on HIV/AIDS (UNAIDS) and the World Health Organization (WHO), is 36.1 million adults and 1.4 million children who were living with HIV at the end of 2000. This is more than 50 percent higher that the figures projected by WHO in 1991 based on the data then available.

Number of people infected during 2000, and the number of deaths...

Fortunately for the US, AIDS deaths declined overall... In the first nine months of last year, 30,700 people in the United States died from AIDS, down 19 Percent from the 37,900 who died in the first nine months of 1995, according to the Centers for Disease Control (CDC). Unfortunately, the improvements are less for African- Americans, woman, Hispanics, heterosexuals and IV drug users.

During 2000, some 5.3 million people were infected with the human immunodeficiency virus (HIV), which causes AIDS. The year also saw 3 million deaths from HIV/AIDS ...

On the continent of Africa, AIDS is now the leading cause of death, in Africa, overtaking malaria as the continent's main killer disease, the United Nations has said.

It said the epidemic was responsible for one in five of all deaths in Africa last year.

Worldwide, the UN said, AIDS is now a bigger killer than any other infectious disease— and the fourth overall cause of death, after heart disease, strokes and respiratory infections, which often affect people in old age.

AIDS more than anywhere else in the world affects the continent of Africa. The UN estimates that more than 11 million people have now died of the disease.

The Caribbean and Latin America

In Latin America an estimated 150,000 adults and children became infected during 2000. By the end of the year, some 1.4 million adults and children in the region were estimated to be living with HIV or AIDS, as compared with 1.3 million at the end of 1999.

Fifteen years ago, AIDS was almost unknown. Currently 33 million people in the world live with HIV. By the end of this year, studies conservatively estimates that 39 million people may be infected - more than all those killed in the Second World War. 1996... International Conference on AIDS held in Vancouver. India declared the country with the largest number of HIV infected people. The joint report of UN AIDS, AIDSCAP and the Harvard School of Public Health presented at Vancouver declared that "evidence suggests an estimate of between 2 and 5 million" HIV infections in India at that moment. This highlights the impact of HIV/AIDS on the economy of India.

Formidable threat

Peter Piot, executive director of the UN AIDS, the body responsible for co-coordinating the fight against AIDS, said. "It is the most formidable disease to confront modern medicine, with the potential to undermine the massive improvements made this century in global health and well being."

He said, "HIV was catastrophic for two reasons: AIDS targets young adults and the number of deaths are accelerating quickly.'

"Even if we stopped HIV today, because of the millions of people now living with the infection, the burden of AIDS will continue to be severely felt."

"This is only the tip of the iceberg," he said.

Millions died

The UN estimates that two million Africans died of AIDS last year. This is well over 80 Percent of the worldwide death toll.

It said the epidemic was responsible for one in five of all deaths in Africa last year.

With the awareness of these alarming statistics, it has been impressed upon me to spread the good news of hope for the hopeless; that is why it bears repeating to include a redacted segment of a previous chapter of my first book here:

The Best Cure for AIDS

AIDS

A disease caused by strains of a virus known as HIV (human immunodeficency virus), that attacks certain white blood cells called T4, or CD4, cells. According to medical science the virus is spread through the exchange of body fluids (primarily semen, blood, and blood products) and can persist in the body for a decade or more without any apparent symptoms.

AZT

Drug used to treat patients infected with the human immunodeficiency virus (HIV), which causes AIDS; also called azidothymidine. It inhibits the virus's ability to reproduce and may decrease the frequency of infection by other diseases, enhancing the lives of HIV-infected patients, but it does not cure AIDS.

Two other drugs that act similarly to AZT: ddI (didanosine or dideoxyinosine) and da4 (stavudine), used to treat patients who do not respond to or cannot tolerate AZT. Another similar-acting drug is ddC (zalcitabine or dideoxycytidine) in combination with AZT.

The disease weakens the body's immune system, allowing other diseases, including Kaposi's sarcoma (otherwise a relatively uncommon and benign form of cancer), Pneumocystis carinii pneumonia, pulmonary tuberculosis, invasive cervical cancer, and encephalitis, to overwhelm the individual.

Very frightening, this is scary stuff! However, there is hope that transcends it. Would you like to hear about it?

To whom it may concern: Allow me to recommend you to the best cure for the AIDS virus, a panacea for all that ails you! In all fairness and honesty, the solution to your problems is the perfect blood transfusion that is safe from the AIDS virus: The Blood Atonement.

Divine Atonement

This Divine atonement can be traced right back to the Garden of Eden when Adam and Eve's sin separated them from their Creator. Who, after He had created man in His own image, and breathed into him the breath of life, man became a living soul, with body and Spirit. Because of sin and disobedience, the only thing that could atone and redeem man back to God his Creator is blood sacrifice of Divine acceptance.

Further evidence of this fact was demonstrated when the blood sacrifice of Able, Adam's first son, was accepted unto God; but the sacrifice of Cain rejected, because it was not a blood sacrifice unto God his Creator!

God continues to demonstrate his love towards us nevertheless.... Je-hovah-ji'reh, through Christ, our redeemer being made the sacrificial Lamb. "The only begotten of the Father, full of grace and truth." "The Lamb of God; slain from before the foundation of the world." "The blood sprinkling that speaketh better things than that of Able." He shed his precious blood on the cross for our sins so that men and women of Adam's fallen race can be redeemed back into His favor.

Oh, what a marvelous plan and act of redeeming love the Father has demonstrated to redeem fallen man. Only Je- hovah-ji'reh, our Creator and provider can deliver this way. Fossil rock or mere mortal, with finite limitations, cannot.

Is there any other who is like the omnipotent Omniscient (All knowing) God who could have made man from the dust of the ground into a living being? Having a soul, Body, and spirit?

Pardon this slight tangent as I aver my faith based on personal experience: I think I can state unequivocally that my faith is impervious to change, due to the fact that there is no other God who can deliver after this sort.... No sculptured work of art and science, *based on the theory of evolution, can create flesh and blood out of the dust of the ground, like God the Creator has done: which I aver with absolute certainty.*

Such a unique act of sovereignty is unparalleled, unmatched, unrivalled and impervious to being duplicated.

Has there ever been a possibility? On the other hand, will there ever be? Whether by means of cloning or artificial insemination that will replicate a perfect species in the form of a human being, then breathe the breath of life into what he has made as flesh and blood from the dust of the ground? The answer to the question is a resounding "no!" to which I aver with absolute certainty.

Let us continue with the discussion of the unique life giving power of blood Atonement!

The word of God is absolute! With God, there is no equal. Neither is there any likeness unto Him. Any attempt made to imitate, or duplicate any act of God's creation; one would have to be able to make something out of nothing.

Therefore, only the true and living God can create something out of nothing. There you have the absolute facts, the authentic proof of creation. By this may all men know! Only the Perfect Blood of the Lamb of God can truly atone for the sins of man; whom He has created, and that is the fact that wins every contest! Let's continue with the subject of AIDS.

Food for Thought for Inquiring Minds

Here is "food for thought" — for all concerned! ... This is a redacted chapter of my first book. We are living in a very fearful time in history where everyone is afraid of the dreaded disease called AIDS.

The transmission of AIDS is through body fluids, primarily semen, blood, and contaminated blood products through the blood stream of the body. To the laypersons not extensively trained in the physiology of the human body, one might ask why through the blood stream. This is what the Bible has to say about it. We read in Leviticus 17:11, the following: "For the life of the flesh is in the blood: and I have given it to you upon the altar to make atonement for your souls, for it is the blood that maketh atonement for the soul."

That is right; the life is in the blood, therefore, if the blood is contaminated, it will eventually destroy the whole body.

For the said reasons, who in his or her right mind would want to mingle with contaminated blood? Think of one person in this world who is dearest to you. No doubt the majority of people would say their mother or their wife or whomever he or she may be. Because of the fear of AIDS in the world today, no one wants to have a questionable transfusion mingled with contaminated blood. Not even if you were aware that that contaminated blood is the blood of your dearest loved one.

However, there is one person, whose blood, not only mingles with my blood, whose blood I am not afraid of catching AIDS from, because it has washed me, cleansed me, and made me whole! That precious blood is none other than the blood of Jesus.

May I say this: In order to save us from the impending wrath of God, let us be cleansed with the blood that can save us, and not destroy us with the AIDS virus, and the ultimate destruction that follows, which is death and hell. "Much more then, being now justified by his blood, we shall be saved from wrath through him" (Romans 5:9).

Because the blood of Christ is perfect in grace and mercy, for the atonement of sin, the apostle Paul reiterates the same proclamation concerning the redemptive power of the blood of the Lamb, as declared above.

In summation:
In this time of Universal Grief...

The perfect formula for such a time as this is the perfect blood transfusion that can heal soul, body, and spirit.

The infallible word of truth, proclaimed this blood to be a panacea, cure for all! There is no fear in this blood! The only fear is found in those who refused to accept its cleansing power to forgive sins.

A Soul is A Terrible Thing to Waste!

CHAPTER 13

How to Deal with the Battle of the Will

The battle of the will is defined in many ways, with each taking on a defined character of its own. For example, a person may have a strong need to do something that is inherently good, but lack the will to it.

Let us take, for example, a person wanting to kick the habit of smoking, but unable to do so on his/her own. For the most part, his willingness may be evident, but the desire for the taste of the narcotic is overwhelming. As a result, failure seems to be the order of the day, rather than his desired goal.

Case in point: I read a story of a woman's husband who was a chain smoker of several packs of cigarettes a day. She was greatly concerned for the health of her husband and rightly so. Each night as he sat asleep in his easy chair in front of the TV set, and after he had gone to bed, she would whisper softly in his ear several times: "Cigarettes cause lung cancer, stop smoking."

One day, after several months had passed and Suzy was about ready to give up this unorthodox procedure, Joe said to her: "I've decided to quit smoking." When she asked him why, he replied, "

I don't really know why. It's just that something inside of me kept saying not to smoke any more, so I am not going to." Several years have passed and her husband has not smoked a single cigarette since then.

The preceding story illustrates how nonscientific methods can remarkably facilitate ones effort in combating the battle of the will to kick the habit of smoking.

How to Stop Smoking Cold Turkey...

The experts give five general techniques for your bad habits. You can put them to work yourself; and they are the following:

(1) You must reach the point where you can no longer tolerate yourself the way you are or the situation the way that it is.

(2) You must be free of your bad habit more than you want to hang onto it.

(3) You must establish tangible and concrete goals to reach, or benefits to achieve.

(4) Do it only one day at a time

That said, and for all good intentioned purposes, there is always the fear factor that is so pervasive in the hearts and minds of men and women everywhere. On the other hand, fear can be one of the biggest motivators in giving up cigarette smoking.

Pros and Cons of Fear

"It is important to remember that fear is always on the opposite side of bold and good desire." You want to smoke, but the fear of cancer, heart attack, bronchitis, asthma, and emphysema must be stronger than your desire for a cigarette. This is one time when fear can be beneficial to you.

For example, a man smoked three to four packs of cigarettes every day until he was 50 years old, even though he may have been a doctor and known better.

Suddenly he wakes up one morning with a tremendous pain in his chest. He feels as if someone has thrown a huge spear through his chest, all the way through and out through his back.

The excruciating pain persisted continually for many days, yet he continued to smoke in spite of it. On a certain day, he made the decision to stop smoking and did just that, because he had finally reached the point that he wanted to quit more than he wanted to smoke. He was scared to death of possible lung cancer. Over 20 years have passed and he has not touched a single cigarette.

The pain in his chest disappeared within days after he quit smoking and has never returned. His lungs are clean and clear. X-rays show them to be as healthy as the lungs of a person who has never smoked. He has more energy and his food tastes better. From this experience, one can clearly see the benefits of not smoking far outweigh the benefits of smoking¾if there are any benefits at all in smoking.

You and your family may also want to kick the habit of smoking. Your doctor might have warned you of an irregular heartbeat because of cigarettes and you want to quit smoking cold turkey because of fear, never to smoke again.

Vanity vs. motivation

Vanity sometimes is a motivating factor in ones decision to do something about maintaining their exquisite beauty.

A person may be a habitual smoker over a number of years, only to find one day, while reading a magazine article, that women who smoke have more wrinkles at 50 than nonsmokers at 70.

Immediately after reading this article, you go to the supermarket and see a little old woman sitting on a bench waiting for the bus. You may describe that woman later. “That woman had more wrinkles than I’ve ever seen. She had wrinkles on top of wrinkles!”

That might motivate you never to smoke another cigarette again because you have witnessed the result of what smoking can do to a person’s body. You are convinced that if smoking makes you look like that, it just isn’t worth sacrificing your exquisite beauty. (On the other hand, the attractiveness of a man’s physique.)

For years, you might have read many articles on the dangerous consequences of smoking and the pitfalls of lung cancer, with no obvious effect. However, one glimpse of what you might look like if you keep on smoking was enough to make you stop cold turkey. In this case, vanity and the fear of losing your salient beauty was a bigger motivator than fear of illness.

Whatever your motivating factor, the experts advise that you list all the benefits you can think of to convince yourself that it is more worthwhile to quit, than it is to continue smoking.

Here is a list of suggested benefits you will receive if you follow the experts advice:

(1) You will not have a hacking smoker’s cough, deleterious to yourself and others as well.

(2) Your lungs will heal very fast and you will not run the risk of cancer, bronchitis, asthma, and emphysema.

(3) Your food will have its natural aroma and taste better because smoking impairs not only your sense of taste, but also your sense of smell

(4) You will reduce the strain on your vascular system and lower your blood pressure, which reduces the risk of crippling stroke.

(5) You will greatly minimize the risk of heart attack.

(6) You will not run the risk of excessive facial wrinkles, an important benefit to consider, for both men and women.

(7) You will save money. Example, a two-pack-a-day- at $5.00! Going up to $6.00! a pack will cost you more than $2000!! a year. That represents a large sum of money.

(8) You will live longer. According to insurance statistics, nonsmokers lifespan is much longer than that of smokers, life will be much more enjoyable as well.

(9) You will be free! One of the biggest¾freedom from addiction, not being bound to bad habits, you have no choice in the matter. The urge to smoke is greater than your willpower not to smoke.

When you are free of the habit, your decision- making ability is greatly enhanced, and that's a wonderful sense of relief.

Now that you are advised of the plethora of benefits to gain when you give up smoking, instead of trying to quit by using willpower of your imagination, program your mind to succeed from these benefits even if you have tried and failed many times before.

"When imagination and willpower work juxtaposed together, and are pulling in the same, direction aimed toward the same goal, an irresistible force is created, which is an important concomitant of success. Success is then inevitable."

CHAPTER 14

How to Deal with Overweight Problems

One of our nation's former talk show hosts watched a comedian imitating him¾as a fat man. The comic had stuffed himself with padding and the famous host could not stand the caricature. Therefore, he went on a diet and exercise program, and soon was able to show off his new slim body to his audience.

Why the change? "The host had hit bottom" the point where he could no longer tolerate himself the way he was. That is when he decided to do something about it.

For many people, the motivating factor in losing excess weight is better health; for others, just as in smoking, it is vanity.

No matter what the motivation, just as in kicking the smoking habit, "Willpower is not the key to success." You must use your God-given imagination to utilize all the possible benefits you can gain and program them into your creative mind so you can lose those unwanted pounds. The experts lists some of the benefits for you as the following:

(1) You will have more energy, more vitality, more pep and go power.

(2) You will no longer be short of breath.

(3) Your complexion will be clear; your hair will shine.

(4) You will be regular without laxatives; your digestion will improve; you will be free from heartburn and acid stomach.

(5) You will not be nervous and high-strung; you will even sleep better.

(6) If you are a woman, people may mistake you for your daughter.

(7) In addition, if you are a woman, you will not have to make any excuse for your figure.

(8) You can be the envy of all your "plump" friends.

(9) You will look and feel five to ten years younger.

(10) Your love life will improve dramatically.

(11) You will run less risk of heart attack.

(12) Your blood pressure will be much lower.

(13) Your circulation will improve markedly.

(14) According to insurance statistics, you will live longer…

(15) Your low, nagging backache will disappear.

(16) Your arthritis and rheumatism will be less painful…

(17) Life will definitely become worth living once again…

Now that is a plethora of benefits you can gain when you get rid of your excess weight. You must use your God- given imagination and program your creative mind with all these benefits that can be yours when you tone down. Then losing weight will become easy for you.

As further motivation, you can program your mind with vivid images just as hundreds of successful weight watchers do. One innovative individual… I will name her Suzy. Scotch taped two pictures of herself to her refrigerator door. One showed what she looked like when she graduated from high school and was a slim 115 pounds. The other was a current one, with her weight at 190 pounds. It took her about six months to get rid of 75 pounds, but she succeeded for what she was motivated by, as she saw what was staring at her from her refrigerator door.

Willpower: will it work for you?

If you rely on your willpower to get rid of your excess weight as Suzy did, your success is not guaranteed. Suzy continued to fight her problem by relying on her own willpower to conquer it.

She wanted to prove to herself that she had the willpower to resist her desire for sweets. She put a box of chocolates on the dining room table and then sat down to stare hungrily at them, vowing to herself not to touch one. Sad to say, she ate the box of candy, which was very pleasing to her aesthetic taste! Her weak willpower could not resist the overwhelming force against her will.

Today she is slim and no longer carrying around her excess fat. She got rid of it after she learned not to use her weak willpower, but to concentrate on the benefits she would gain by loosing her excess weight.

Using your creative mind to get rid of bad habits

"When you fight your problem of excess fat, or any other problems you have, say the experts; the way Suzy did: when you antagonize any unfavorable situation and allow it to tempt you, you are programming your minds with wrong goals. In doing that, you simply give your problem more power over you. You deplete your own power to gain victory to that same extent: Many times, especially at first glance, resistance seems to be the only way out of your dilemma."

You might ask, what is willpower? "It is useful in only one way, making the initial decision to change, whether that change is to lose weight, stop smoking, quit drinking, put things off, get rid of a bad temper, or whatever your bad habits are. Once the decision is made with willpower, then you must use your imagination to program your creative mind with the benefits you will receive so you can make that decision to make willpower stick."

As stated earlier, when imagination and willpower are in agreement with each other, when they are harmoniously juxtaposed pulling, in the same direction, an irresistible force is created, which is an important component of success.

As with smoking and many other bad habits, sometimes what vanity, fear and other maladies might lead to, is enough motivating factor to change bad habits in an individual life.

A personal experience

This is a personal note of my experience with vanity consciousness and my response over a comment made by a barber shop guest about a bulging abdomen I had at that time, which I personally did not see as a problem, despite my wife's occasional reference to that affect.

Many years ago, I developed a bad habit of eating ice cream and donuts after dinner at night, sometimes before bedtime. That type of nocturnal bad habit resulted in me having a slight bulging stomach. Once I was sitting in a barbershop waiting for my haircut. This person made disparaging remarks about my stomach, and asked if I was pregnant, which led to a series of crude laughter.

Those offensive remarks lacerated my pride and motivated me to take pride in myself by adhering to proper nutritional diet, and to maintain my masculinity as the Creator has intended me, not to confuse anyone of my gender.

As stated previously: Vanity can sometimes-motivate one into making radical changes for a better life-style and eating habits. I maintain a steady weight of approximately 185 lbs for many years since that embarrassing experience that lacerated my pride many years ago. Since then, I practice proper eating habits by not eating donuts and ice cream after meals, especially at night.

In summation on the subject of willpower...

...When imagination and willpower are harmoniously juxtaposed, an irresistible force is created which is an important component of success. Unfortunately for those, whose lives we mourn on September 11, the stalwart firefighters, police officers, and good samaratans who gave their lives in order to save others: Though you're not here with us, your inviolable legacy of true altruism has enriched us all.

United We Stand Against the Access of Evil ...

Simeon W. Johnson

www.ingramcontent.com/pod-product-compliance
Lightning Source LLC
LaVergne TN
LVHW050917210926
848482LV00012B/480